This user-friendly handbook is intended to help the busy physician with that first critical step in clinical diagnosis: how to determine that this is an inherited metabolic disease, and where does one go from here to establish a diagnosis. The well-illustrated text is organized around the clinical presentation of the disease, to facilitate rapid diagnosis, and then clearly explains how to go about identifying the underlying biochemical and genetic lesion. It will therefore complement those more traditional textbooks of metabolic disease which are organized biochemically. The book is intended to serve as an entrance to the discipline, to help nonexpert physicians and advanced medical trainees to overcome the intimidation they are accustomed to experiencing when dealing with metabolic problems.

A clinical guide to inherited
metabolic diseases

A clinical guide to inherited metabolic diseases

Joe T.R. Clarke
M.D., Ph.D., FRCP(C), FCCMG
Department of Paediatrics University of Toronto and
Division of Clinical Genetics, The Hospital for Sick Children

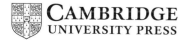

CAMBRIDGE
UNIVERSITY PRESS

Coventry University

Published by the Press Syndicate of the University of Cambridge
The Pitt Building, Trumpington Street, Cambridge CB2 1RP
40 West 20th Street, New York, NY 10011-4211, USA
10 Stamford Road, Oakleigh, Melbourne 3166, Australia

© Cambridge University Press 1996

First published 1996

Printed in Great Britain at the University Press, Cambridge

Typeset in Garamond $10\frac{1}{4}/13$

A catalogue record for this book is available from the British Library

Library of Congress cataloguing in publication data

Clarke, Joe T. R.
A clinical guide to inherited metabolic diseases / Joe T. R.
Clarke.
     p.   cm.
Includes bibliographical references.
ISBN 0-521-48064-7 (hardback). – ISBN 0-521-48524-X (pbk.)
1. Metabolism, Inborne errors of. I. Title.
[DNLM: 1. Metabolism, Inborn Errors – diagnosis. 2. Metabolism,
Inborn Errors – genetics. 3. Diagnosis, Differential. 4. Diagnosis,
Laboratory. 5. Metabolism, Inborn Errors – therapy. WD 205 C598c
1996]
RC627.8.C53 1996
616.3'9042 – dc20 96–10270 CIP
DNLM/DLC
for Library of Congress

ISBN 0 521 48064 7 hardback
ISBN 0 521 48524 X paperback

Dedicated to the memory of my late father

THOMAS ROY CLARKE

MD, FRCS(C), FRCOG

a consummate clinician in his day.

Contents

Preface

Over the past three decades, enormous strides have been made in the recognition and understanding of diseases caused by genetic defects of specific enzymes and transport proteins. Most of the progress has been made through basic research employing new and rapidly evolving concepts and techniques in biochemical and molecular genetics. The attention of most investigators in the field has quite naturally focused on how specific point defects in metabolism cause disease. In the process, we have learned a great deal about normal intermediary metabolism in addition to how specific mutations produce metabolic disease. Being able to describe to medical students and clinical trainees in medicine how the signs and symptoms of specific diseases can be explained by what is known about the metabolic effects of the relevant genetic defects has been exciting and richly rewarding. It is supported by a number of excellent texts on the subject. The monumental text, *The Metabolic and Molecular Bases of Inherited Disease*, edited by Charles Scriver and his colleagues, provides the finest single-source overview of what is known about the relationship between mutation and inherited metabolic disease. It has been, and I expect it will remain for some time, the standard text on the subject.

Progress on the reverse process, on how to identify individuals with specific inborn errors of metabolism on the basis of signs and symptoms of disease, has been slower. The trouble is that the human appears to have a limited repetoire of ways to respond to insult, with the result that the clinical features of many inherited metabolic diseases tend to be more alike than they are different. What is even more frustrating to medical trainees or general physicians with little experience in the area is that the clinical presentation of many inherited metabolic diseases may be superficially indistinguishable from that of acquired conditions, such as infections or intoxications, which are much more common than diseases caused by inborn errors of metabolism. Patients presenting with symptoms of disease do not come bearing a label indicating that they have an inborn error of metabolism. And even when told that a patient has an inherited metabolic disease, most medical trainees and physicians who are not specialists in the field have difficulty figuring out how to proceed to identify the basic metabolic defect on the basis of the clinical manifestations of the disease.

Some clinicians have attempted to provide guidance through this diagnostic labyrinth, and there are some good review articles on various aspects of the subject. In this regard, Jean-Marie Saudubray has made important contributions. An indication of the difficulty of the undertaking is revealed by the disclaimer made by the editors regarding the chapter on clinical phenotypes and diagnostic algorithms provided by Saudubray and Charpentier for *The Metabolic and Molecular Bases of Inherited Disease*. For years, I have been employing similar approaches to teaching pediatrics residents the fundamentals of the discipline of metabolic genetics. This book is a distillation of some of the basic principles employed in that approach.

The purpose of this book is to provide some guidelines for the recognition of genetic metabolic diseases on the basis of their clinical presentation, and how to go about identifying the underlying biochemical and genetic lesion. It is intended to supplement, not replace, existing texts on inherited metabolic diseases which are organized biochemically. It is organized according to clinical presentation of disease. The reader is guided through an analysis of the clinical findings and the relevant basic biochemistry and physiology in an approach to differential diagnosis that helps in guiding laboratory investigation. It is not intended to be an exhaustive compendium of all inherited metabolic diseases, a task well beyond the intended goal of the work. Instead, the concentration throughout is on a clinical approach to diagnostic problem solving that is founded on principles of pathophysiology using descriptions of specific diseases heuristically to make the point. This book is intended to serve as an entrance to the discipline. With the confidence gained, the nonexpert clinician may be surprised by how quickly things begin to come together and how stimulating the practice of metabolic genetics can be.

The first chapter summarizes some basic principles of genetics and metabolism relevant to the management of inherited metabolic diseases in general. It includes a brief overview of mendelian genetics, an introduction to some general principles of metabolism as they relate to inherited metabolic diseases, and some discussion of common causes of diagnostic confusion. The next seven chapters deal with with genetic metabolic presentations or 'syndromes', constellations of clinical findings commonly encountered in patients presenting with inherited metabolic diseases. The 'syndromes' include neurologic syndrome, hepatic syndrome, metabolic acidosis, cardiac syndromes, storage syndrome and dysmorphology, the positive PKU (phenylketonuria) screening test (arguably one of the commonest indications for genetic metabolic investigation), and acute metabolic illness presenting in the newborn period. One might well have added other chapters, like 'skin syndrome' or 'eye syndrome', in order to discuss inherited metabolic diseases presenting primarily as dermatologic or ocular disease. Therein lies one of the problems with this clinical discipline: no tissue or organ is spared when it comes to inherited metabolic diseases. To include every way in which they may present would vitiate the whole purpose of this book by creating the mass of arcane detail that makes the discipline so daunting in the first place. The 'syndromes' selected for discussion are common ways for inherited metabolic diseases to present; they are, by no means, the only ways.

Some may wonder at the decision to devote an entire chapter to PKU. First, it is historically important. In two critical ways it differed from the conditions that led to Garrod's initial concept of inborn error of metabolism: it was the first inborn error of metabolism to be discovered in which the clinical consequences of the metabolic defect can be devastating, and treatment by environmental manipulation was shown to be dramatically effective in preventing the severe mental retardation associated with it. It is still probably the most common autosomal recessive inborn error of metabolism with the capacity to cause severe, preventable disease in humans. Yet, many clinicians will have had little first-hand experience managing it because the disease is not associated with acute illness requiring frequent or extended hospitalization. Virtually all treatment is carried out on an ambulatory basis at home, with relatively infrequent visits to the hospital or clinic. Secondly, including a chapter on PKU (Chapter 3) provides an opportunity to introduce a discussion of genetic screening. Over the years, the success of newborn PKU screening programs has spawned other attempts to duplicate the experience by applying the same principles to other conditions. This has led to the development of guidelines for genetic screening which are now widely accepted as a model for the evaluation of genetic screening programs in general. The chapter on PKU provides a platform for a brief discussion of these principles of genetic screening which are bound to become increasingly important as proposals for the introduction of screening for other genetic conditions proliferate.

Chapter 9 contains a discussion of diagnostic laboratory issues related to the investigation of possible inherited metabolic diseases. It is intended to provide the clinician with a feel for what is done in the laboratory to test his or her diagnostic hypotheses, and what the limitations are on interpretation of laboratory results. The clinical laboratory is a critical part of the diagnostic armamentarium available to the clinician faced with a possible inherited metabolic disease. The need to be familiar with some of the workings of this indispensable tool would seem to be obvious.

The final chapter provides an overview of contemporary treatment of inherited metabolic diseases. It is organized according to principles of management with specific examples provided to flesh it out. What is presented is included for heuristic purposes, not as a prescription for treatment of any specific disease or situation. The treatment of inherited metabolic diseases is evolving rapidly, and any of the examples of treatment that are currently acceptable may have changed by the time this book is published.

A number of people contributed over the years to the preparation of this book, some of them unaware at the time of the profound influence they had on my thinking. Although many of the ideas contained here can be traced to them, I assume full responsibility for the manner in which they are presented and, in particular, for any errors. I am particularly indebted to Sandy Lowden, whose influence on me, when I was a resident in pediatrics and subsequently, completely altered the direction of my career. I am grateful to my colleagues, Rod McInnes, Annette Feigenbaum, Bill Hanley, Brian Robinson, Ingrid Tein, and Geof Sherwood. However, perhaps the most important group to be acknowledged are the residents and fellows who have rotated through the genetic metabolic service at the Hospital for Sick Children over the years and stimulated me to think in ways that ultimately forged my own approach to inherited metabolic diseases. John Christodoulou, Mohammed Abdul-Jabbar, and Margaret Nowaczyk deserve special mention for continually pressing me to think carefully and clearly about our patients and the innumerable diagnostic problems we tackled together.

I am indebted to many colleagues for providing material for the figures in the book: Jim Phillips provided the superb electron micrographs of the liver, and Venita Jay supplied the electron micrographs of conjunctival epithelium and the photomicrograph of muscle. Susan Blaser provided photographs of the neuroimaging studies; Annette Poon provided a photograph showing Alder-Reilly bodies in leukocytes; and Paul Babyn provided radiographs showing Gaucher disease in the lower limbs. I am grateful to Professor Dr. Jaak Jaeken and Professor Dr. Georg Hoffmann for permission to publish photographs of their patients with carbohydrate-deficient glycoprotein syndrome and mevalonic aciduria, respectively.

A number of colleagues and associates read various parts of the manuscript and offered suggestions which have materially improved the book. Margaret Nowaczyk, Annette Feigenbaum, Denis Lehotay, Debbie Terespolsky, Bill Hanley, and Eve Roberts each read and commented on one or more chapters.

My secretary, Nancy Leung, showed a genius for anticipating my needs and performing a myriad of jobs that needed to be done in order to finish the manuscript and at the same time running a busy office.

My wife, Cathy, provided moral support and, more importantly, tolerated my abiding commitment to this project at the expense of her own needs.

J. T. R. Clarke
Toronto

1

General principles

Introduction

In his 1908 address to the Royal College of Physicians of London, Sir Archibald Garrod coined the expression *inborn error of metabolism* to describe a group of disorders – alkaptonuria, benign pentosuria, albinism, and cystinuria – apparently caused by point defects in the metabolism of simple intermediary metabolites, like amino acids and monosaccharides. He noted that each was a life-long condition, not significantly affected by treatment; that each was transmitted as a recessive trait within families in a way predictable by Mendel's laws of inheritance; and that each was relatively benign. Following Følling's discovery of phenylketonuria (PKU) in 1934, the concept underwent a major change, particularly with respect to its relationship with disease. PKU was shown to be caused by a recessively inherited point defect in the conversion of phenylalanine to tyrosine in the liver. However, unlike Garrod's original four inborn errors of metabolism, PKU was far from benign – it was associated with a particularly severe form of mental retardation. Moreover, although the metabolic defect was 'inborn' and life-long, the associated mental retardation could be prevented by treatment with dietary phenylalanine restriction.

The discovery of PKU sparked the search for other clinically significant inborn errors of metabolism. The number of disorders that have been attributed to inherited point defects in metabolism now exceeds 400 (see Scriver *et al.*, 1995). While they are individually rare, they collectively account for a significant proportion of illness, particularly in children. They present clinically in a wide variety of ways, involving virtually any organ or tissue of the body, and accurate diagnosis is important both for treatment and for the prevention of disease in other family members.

The purpose of this book is to provide a framework of principles to help clinicians recognize when an illness might be caused by an inborn error of metabolism. It presents a problem-oriented clinical approach to determining the type of metabolic defect involved and what investigation is needed to establish a specific diagnosis.

Some general metabolic concepts

Metabolism is the sum total of all the chemical reactions that occur as part of the continuing process of breakdown and renewal in the body. Enzymes play an indispensible role in facilitating the process by serving as catalysts in the conversion of one chemical (metabolite) to another, often extracting the energy required for the reaction from a suitable high-energy source, such as ATP. All enzymes have at least two types of physico-chemical domains: one or more substrate-binding domains, and at least one catalytic domain. The various ways that mutations might affect enzyme activity break down into two general categories: (1) There may not be enough enzyme available to the reaction, owing to a defect in enzyme production or abnormally rapid breakdown of any enzyme produced. (2) Alternatively, the mutation might impair the activity of the enzyme without affecting the amount of enzyme protein.

The rapid transport of metabolites across cellular and subcellular membranes is facilitated in many cases by specific transport proteins which function like enzymes. This means that the process is susceptible to genetic mutations affecting the amount or function of the transporter in exactly the same way that mutation affects the activities of enzymes, and with similar consequences.

Mutations may affect gene products in many ways. The coding sequences of most structural genes are comprised of at least a few thousand nucleotides, and the potential for mutation-generated variations in structure is vast. In the same way, the effects of mutation also vary tremendously. At one extreme, some mutations may totally disrupt the production of any gene product, resulting in severe disease. Whereas, other mutations might have no effect whatsoever apart from a functionally silent change in the nucleotide sequence of the gene. The relationship between genotype and disease phenotype is complex. Severe mutations are generally associated with clinically severe disease, and the disease phenotype among different affected individuals tends to be very similar. Structurally more subtle mutations, such as those resulting in single amino acid substitutions, are often associated with milder disease phenotypes. However, the disease phenotype often varies markedly between different affected individuals, even within the same family, a reminder that the expression of any genetic information, including disease-causing mutations, is influenced by other genes (gene–gene interactions) and by environmental factors (gene–environment interactions).

Disease results from point defects in metabolism

The signs and symptoms of disease in patients with inborn errors of metabolism

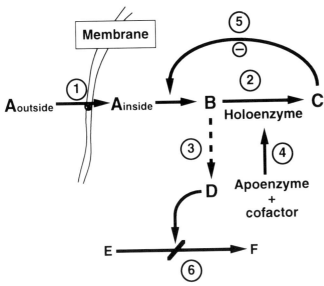

Fig. 1.1. The primary consequences of inborn errors of metabolism. The figure shows diagrammatically the various possible mutation-sensitive defects affecting the compartmentalization and metabolism of Compound A. **1**, transporter-mediated movement of A from one compartment to another; **2**, defect in the conversion of B to C; **3**, increased conversion of B to D caused by accumulation of B; **4**, defect in the interaction between an apoenzyme and an obligatory cofactor; **5**, decreased feedback inhibition of the conversion of A_{in} to B as a result of deficiency of C; and **6**, secondary inhibition of the conversion of E to F caused by accumulation of D.

are the result of metabolic disturbances caused by deficiency of some catalytic or transport protein. Figure 1.1 shows schematically the relationship between various types of defects and their pathophysiologically and diagnostically important consequences.

Accumulation of substrate

Accumulation of the substrate of a mutant enzyme is an important cause of disease in many inborn errors of metabolism, particularly those involving strictly degradative processes. Some examples are shown in Table 1.1.

Accumulation of substrate is also diagnostically important. Specific diagnosis often follows quickly after identification of the accumulation of metabolites proximal to an enzyme defect, particularly among inborn errors of water-soluble substrates. This is generally true, for example, of the amino acidopathies and

Table 1.1. *Some examples of inborn errors of metabolism in which symptoms of disease are the result of substrate accumulation.*

Disease	Metabolic defect	Accumulating substrate	Main clinical findings
Tay-Sachs disease	β-Hexosaminidase A deficiency	GM2 ganglioside in brain	Cerebral neurodegeneration
OTC deficiency	OTC deficiency	Ammonium	Acute encephalopathy
Methylmalonic acidemia	Methylmalonyl-CoA mutase deficiency	Methylmalonic acid	Metabolic acidosis
PKU	Phenylalanine hydroxylase deficiency	Phenylalanine	Progressive mental retardation
Hurler disease	α-L-Iduronidase deficiency	Dermatan and heparan sulfates	Unusual facies, skeletal abnormalities, progressive mental retardation
Cystinuria	Dibasic amino acid transport defect in kidney	Cystine in urine	Recurrent obstructive uropathy
Hepatorenal tyrosinemia	Fumarylacetoacetase deficiency	Fumarylacetoacetate and maleylacetoacetate	Acute hepatocellular dysfunction, cirrhosis, rickets

Note: Abbreviations: OTC, ornithine transcarbamylase; PKU, phenylketonuria.

organic acidopathies, in which accumulation of substrate throughout the body is often massive, and is reflected by changes in plasma and urine.

In inborn errors of metabolism involving water-insoluble substrates, such as complex lipids, accumulation of the immediate substrate of the mutant enzyme is also important in the pathophysiology of disease. However, accumulation of the compounds is often limited to single tissues or organs, such as brain, which are relatively inaccessible. Moreover, chemical isolation and identification of the metabolites is often cumbersome, requiring laboratory expertise that is not routinely available.

In other disorders, such as the mucopolysaccharide storage diseases, the accumulation of substrate is a major factor in the pathophysiology of disease. However, because the metabolism of the substrate requires the participation of a number of different enzymes, any of which may be deficient as a result of mutation, the demonstration of accumulation is diagnostically important only to the extent that it indicates a class of disorders, not one specific disease. The demonstration of mucopolysaccharide accumulation is important as a screening test for inherited defects in mucopolysaccharide metabolism. However, the metabolism of the individual mucopolysaccharides involves 10 or more genetically distinct lysosomal enzymes, and accumulation of the same mucopolysaccharide may occur as a consequence of deficiency of any one of the enzymes. Specific diagnosis in these disorders requires the demonstration of the specific enzyme deficiency in appropriate tissues, such as peripheral blood leukocytes or cultured skin fibroblasts.

Accumulation of a normally minor metabolite

In some disorders, the primary cause of disease is accumulation of a normally minor metabolite, produced in excess by a reaction that is usually of trivial metabolic importance. The cataracts occurring in patients with untreated *galactosemia* occur as a result of accumulation of the sugar alcohol, galactitol, a normally minor metabolite of galactose. In another example, accumulation of the normally minor complex lipid metabolite, psychosine, in the brain of infants with *Krabbe globoid cell leukodystrophy* excites a subacute inflammatory reaction, manifested by appearance in the brain of multinucleated giant cells, called globoid cells. It also causes rapid, severe demyelination, out of proportion to the accumulation of galactocerebroside, the immediate precursor of the defective enzyme.

Table 1.2. *Some examples of inborn errors of metabolism in which symptoms of disease are the result of product deficiency.*

Disease	Metabolic defect	Product deficiency	Main clinical findings
Vitamin D dependency	25-Hydroxycholecalciferol-1α-hydroxylase deficiency	1α, 25-Dihydroxycholecalciferol	Rickets
Hartnup disease	Neutral amino acid transport defect	Niacinamide	Pellagra-like condition
Lysinuric protein intolerance	Dibasic amino acid transport defect	Ornithine	Recurrent hyperammonemia
Hereditary thrombophilia	Protein C defect	Protein C (physiologic anticoagulant)	Recurrent thrombophlebitis
Transcobalamin II deficiency	Transcobalamin II defect	Vitamin B_{12}	Megaloblastic anemia
Congenital hypothyroidism	Various defects in thyroid hormone biosynthesis	Thyroid hormone	Cretinism; goitre
X-linked hypophosphatemic rickets	Renal phosphate transport defect	Phosphate	Rickets

Deficiency of product

Deficiency of the product of a specific reaction is another primary consequence of many inherited metabolic diseases. The extent to which it contributes to disease depends on the metabolic importance of the product. For example, most of the pathologic consequences of defects of biosynthesis are traceable to a deficiency of the product of the relevant reaction – in these cases substrate accumulation plays little or no role in the development of disease. Table 1.2 shows a list of some conditions in which symptoms are the result of a deficiency of the product of some enzymic reaction or transport process.

Among the inborn errors of amino acid biosynthesis, the signs of disease are often the combined result of substrate accumulation and product deficiency. For example, in the urea cycle disorder, *argininosuccinic aciduria*, the defect in the conversion of argininosuccinic acid to arginine causes arginine deficiency, and this, in turn, results in a deficiency of ornithine. Depletion of intramitochondrial ornithine causes accumulation of carbamylphosphate and ammonia resulting in marked hyperammonemic encephalopathy. The importance of arginine deficiency in the pathophysiology of the encephalopathy is shown by the dramatic response to therapeutic administration of a single large dose of arginine (4 mmoles/kg given intravenously).

Deficiency of the products of reactions is important in two other situations common among the inborn errors of metabolism. One of these could be regarded as the result of a *metabolic steal*, a term introduced by Alf Slonin to explain the occurrence of myopathy in some patients with glycogen storage disease due to debrancher enzyme deficiency. Slonin postulated that increased gluconeogenesis in patients with the disease causes accelerated muscle protein breakdown as free amino acids are diverted from protein biosynthesis to gluconeogenesis in an effort to maintain the blood glucose in the face of impaired glycogen breakdown. Another example of the consequences of a metabolic steal is the occurrence of hypoglycemia in patients with hereditary defects in fatty acid oxidation. The over-utilization of glucose and resulting hypoglycemia is a consequence of the inability to meet energy requirements by fatty acid oxidation.

Another mechanism by which a metabolic defect causes symptoms because of deficiency or inaccessibility of a product might be called *metabolic sequestration*. Transport defects caused by mutations affecting proteins involved in carrier-mediated transport often produce disease through a failure of the transfer of a metabolite from one subcellular compartment to another. The *HHH syndrome*, named for the associated hyperammonemia, hyperornithinemia, and homocitrullinemia, is caused by a defect in the transport of the amino acid, ornithine, into the mitochondria. The resulting intramitochondrial ornithine deficiency

Table 1.3. *Some examples of inborn errors of metabolism in which secondary metabolic defects play a prominent role in the production of symptoms of disease.*

Disease	Metabolic defect	Secondary metabolic abnormalities	Main clinical findings
CAH	21-Hydroxylase deficiency	Aldosterone and cortisol deficiency	Addisonian crisis; virilization of females
GSD type I	Glucose-6-phosphatase deficiency	Lactic acidosis; hyperuricemia; hypertriglyceridemia	Massive hepatomegaly; hypoglycemia; failure to thrive
HFI	Fructose-1-phosphate aldolase deficiency	Lactic acidosis; hypoglycemia; hyperuricemia; hypophosphatemia	Severe metabolic acidosis; hypoglycemia
Methylmalonic acidemia	Methylmalonyl-CoA mutase deficiency	Hyperammonemia; hyperglycinemia	Acute encephalopathy; metabolic acidosis
HHH syndrome	Ornithine transport defect	Homocitrullinemia	Hyperammonemic encephalopathy
OTC deficiency	OTC deficiency	Orotic aciduria	Hyperammonemic encephalopathy
Abetalipoproteinemia	Apolipoprotein B deficiency	Malabsorption of vitamin E	Spinocerebellar degeneration

Note: Abbreviations: CAH, congenital adrenal hyperplasia; GSD, glycogen storage disease; HFI, hereditary fructose intolerance; OTC, ornithine transcarbamylase; HHH, hyperammonemia-hyperornithinemia-homocitrullinemia.

causes accumulation of carbamylphosphate and ammonia, ultimately causing hyperammonemic encephalopathy in a manner similar to that causing the hyperammonemia in argininosuccinic aciduria described above.

Secondary metabolic phenomena

Because of the close interrelationship between the various processes comprising intermediary metabolism, enzyme deficiencies or transport defects inevitably have effects beyond the immediate changes in the concentrations of substrate and product of any particular reaction. These secondary metabolic phenomena often cause diagnostic confusion. For example, *ketotic hyperglycinemia* was initially thought to be a primary disorder of glycine metabolism. However, subsequent studies showed that the hyperglycinemia was actually a secondary metabolic phenomenon in patients with a primary defect of propionic acid metabolism. Furthermore, the acute forms of other organic acidopathies, such as *methyl-malonic acidemia* (see Chapter 4), were also found to be associated with marked accumulation of glycine, severe ketoacidosis, and hyperammonemia, all the result of secondary metabolic effects of organic acid or organic acyl-CoA accumulation. Table 1.3 lists some examples of potentially confusing secondary metabolic responses to point defects in metabolism.

Inborn errors of metabolism are inherited

Determination of the pattern of inheritance of a condition is often helpful in making a diagnosis of genetic disease, and it provides the foundation for genetic counselling. The most important information required for establishing the pattern of inheritance is a family history covering at least three generations of relations.

Autosomal recessive disorders

Most of the inherited metabolic diseases recognized today are inherited in the same manner as Garrod's original inborn errors of metabolism: they are Mendelian, single-gene defects, transmitted in an autosomal recessive manner. Disease expression requires that an individual be homozygous for significant, though not necessarily the same, mutations in the same gene. Theoretically, homozygosity may arise as a result of one of the following:

* simultaneous mutations occurring in the same gene in the same individual at the same time;
* inheritance of one mutation and generation of the second by new mutation;
* inheritance of both mutations from heterozygous parents;

- inheritance of two copies of a mutation from one heterozygous parent as a result of the phenomenon of uniparental isodisomy.

The mutation rate for most human genes is estimated to be extremely low (of the order of 10^{-5} to 10^{-6} mutations per locus per generation), and the probability of homozygosity occurring as a result of simultaneous mutations at the same locus is so small that it can be ignored. Similarly, the possibility of a new mutation occurring in the same gene as that bearing an inherited recessive mutation on the homologous chromosome is extremely low, and it too is generally ignored. The incidence of uniparental isodisomy is not known, but it is probably rare. For the purposes of genetic counselling, the parents of individuals who are homozygous for autosomal recessive disorders are considered to be obligate heterozygotes for disease-causing mutant alleles in the same gene.

Most individuals with autosomal recessive inherited metabolic diseases have no family history of the disorder. However, the occurrence of a similar disorder in a sibling or in a cousin should raise the suspicion that the condition is not only hereditary, but that it is transmitted as an autosomal recessive disorder. Obtaining this information may be difficult because the occurrence of serious disease in children, particularly if it is associated with mental retardation, early infant death, or physical deformities, may be concealed by the family out of shame or simply forgotten.

Consanguinity increases the likelihood that an inherited disorder is autosomal recessive because it increases the probability that both parents of a child are carriers of a rare recessive mutation. As a rule, the rarer it is, the more likely the occurrence an autosomal recessive condition will be affected by inbreeding. For some very rare disorders, the frequency of consanguinity of the parents of affected individuals is as high as 30–40%. Geographic or socio-cultural isolation of relatively small and demographically stable communities increases the risk of inadvertent inbreeding, no doubt contributing to the high frequency of certain diseases in specific ethnic groups. When considering the possibility that the disease in an individual may be the result of an autosomal recessive mutation, the family history should include specific questions to assess the possibility of parental consanguinity. Simply asking the parents if they are related will often reveal the fact. The origins of the parents are also important. The possibility of consanguinity is increased, for example, if the parents of a patient both come from a small village with a history of population stability, and if relatives on the maternal and paternal sides of the family share the same surname.

The increased incidence of a specific inborn error of metabolism in a demographically isolated and stable population as a result of the introduction of

Table 1.4. *Some examples of inborn errors of metabolism occurring in high frequency among specific ethnic groups.*

Disorder	Ethnic group	Estimated incidence (per 100,000 births)
Tay-Sachs disease	Ashkenazi Jews	33*
Gaucher disease, type I	Ashkenazi Jews	100
Hepatorenal tyrosinemia	French-Canadians (Saguenay-Lac Saint-Jean region)	54*
Porphyria variegata	South African (white)	300
Congenital adrenal hyperplasia	Yupik Eskimos	200
Phenylketonuria (PKU)	Turkish	38.5
	Yemenite Jews	19
	Ashkenazi Jews	5
Glutaric aciduria, type I	Ojibway Indians (Canada)	>50†
	Swedish	3.3
Maple syrup urine disease	Mennonites (Pennsylvania)	568

Note: * Before the introduction of prenatal diagnosis to prevent the condition.
† Estimated.
Source: Data derived in part from Weatherall, D.J. (1991) and Scriver et al. (1995).

the mutation by a founding member of the population is called a *founder effect.* The high incidences of certain rare inherited metabolic disorders in specific ethnic groups or communities are well known examples of a putative founder effect, though the role of an element of environmental selection favoring heterozygotes has not been eliminated in some cases. Some examples of inborn errors of metabolism occurring in particularly high frequency in specfic ethnic groups are shown in Table 1.4.

X-linked recessive disorders

In males, it only takes one mutation of a gene on the X chromosome to produce disease. Unlike autosomal recessive disorders, in which the contribution of new mutations to the occurrence of disease in individuals is negligible, about a third of males with X-linked recessive diseases are born to mothers who are *not* carriers of the mutation: the boys are affected as a result of new mutations. For the purposes of genetic counselling, once the medical diagnosis has been confirmed and the possibilities of autosomal recessive and nongenetic phenocopies have been eliminated, it is critical to determine whether the disease caused by an X-linked recessive mutation developed as a result of inheritance of the mutation,

Table 1.5. *Some mechanisms of autosomal dominance.*

Mechanism	Gene product	Disease example
Abnormal assembly of the subunits of a multimeric protein	Fibrillin	Marfan syndrome
Abnormal interaction between the subunits of multimeric protein	Hemoglobin	Hemoglobin M disease
Derepression of rate-limiting enzyme activity	Porphobilinogen deaminase	Acute intermittent porphyria (derepression of δ-aminolevulinic acid dehydratase)
Cell receptor defects	LDL-receptor	Familial hypercholesterolemia (derepression of HMG-CoA reductase)
Cell membrane defects	Spectrin	Hereditary spherocytosis
Deposition of an abnormal structural protein	Transthyretin	Hereditary amyloidosis
Somatic cell mutation coupled with inheritance of a recessive gene	pp110^{RB}	Retinoblastoma

Note: Abbreviations: LDL, low-density lipoprotein; HMG-CoA, 3-hydroxy-3-methylglutaryl-CoA.

or as a result of a new mutation. The family history is particularly important in this situation. The likelihood that the mother of a boy with an X-linked recessive disease inherited the mutation from her own mother can be estimated from the number of healthy male relatives she has related to her through her mother and sisters. For example, the mother of a boy with *Hunter disease* (MPS II), an X-linked recessive mucopolysaccharide storage disease, is unlikely to have inherited the mutation from her own mother if she has a large number of healthy brothers and nephews (i.e., sons of her sisters). The larger the number of healthy male relatives, the more likely the affected boy has the disease as a result of a new mutation, and the lower the risk that his mother is a carrier of Hunter disease. It is a mistake to assume automatically that a woman is a carrier of an X-linked disease if she has a son affected with it. But, if a woman has two affected sons, or she has an affected brother as well as an affected son, she is regarded as an obligate carrier of the disease-causing mutation. It also follows that all the female offspring of a man affected with an X-linked recessive disorder are obligate carriers of the disease; in contrast, none of his sons would be affected because male to male transmission of X-linked recessive conditions does not occur.

Autosomal dominant disorders

Although autosomal dominant mutations are common causes of genetic disease in humans, they contribute relatively little to the sum total of inherited metabolic disorders. This is probably because, with a few exceptions, most inherited metabolic diseases are caused by abnormalities in enzymes or transport proteins that are not involved in the types of interactions or processes required to produce dominance (Table 1.5).

Autosomal dominant inheritance is characterized by:

- every affected individual has an affected parent (unless the individual has the disease as a result of a new mutation, or the mutation is non-penetrant);
- on average half of the offspring of an affected individual will also be affected with the disease;
- unaffected children of an affected individual will themselves have only unaffected children (assuming penetrance is complete);
- males and females are equally represented among affected members of the kindred;
- transmission of the condition occurs vertically through successive generations, unless the condition impairs reproduction.

Because only one mutation is required to cause disease, new mutations contribute significantly to the incidence of autosomal dominant disorders. The

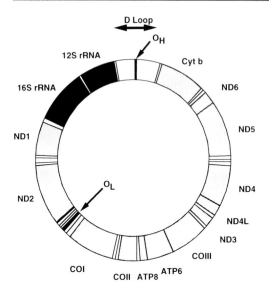

Fig. 1.2. The human mitochondrial genome.
The human mitochondrial genome is encoded in a double-stranded, circular
mtDNA molecule. The figure shows the identity and relative locations of
mitochondrial genes.

rate of spontaneous mutation, and hence the likelihood in any particular
situation that disease is due to spontaneous mutation, varies from one disease to
another.

Mitochondrial inheritance

Each mitochondrion in every cell contains several copies of a small, circular,
double-stranded DNA molecule (mtDNA) containing genes coding for the
production of ribosomal RNA and the various tRNAs necessary for mitochondrial protein biosynthesis, and for the production of some of the proteins
involved in mitochondrial electron transport (Figure 1.2). The mitochondrial
genome consists of 16,569 basepairs, comprising 5523 codons, coding for the
production of 37 gene products.

The vast majority of mitochondrial proteins, including most of the proteins of
subunits involved in electron transport (see Table 4.5), are coded by nuclear
genes. Mutations of these genes cause diseases transmitted as autosomal recessive
disorders. As in the case of other autosomal recessive conditions, the disease
phenotype of various affected individuals in the same family tends to be very
similar.

The situation is quite different with regard to the pattern of inheritance and clinical expression of disease caused by mtDNA mutations. The mitochondria in the cells of each individual are derived at the time of conception from the mitochondria in the cytoplasm of the ovum; the mitochondria and mtDNA of the sperm are lost during the process of fertilization. It follows that mtDNA mutations are also inherited only from the mother. When multiple members of a family are affected with a condition because of inheritance of a mtDNA mutation, the pattern of inheritance is quite specific:

- all the offspring of a woman carrying a mtDNA mutation can generally be shown to have inherited the mutation, whether they are clinically affected with disease or not;
- the phenotypic expression of disease in different individuals who have inherited mtDNA mutations is often highly variable, both in terms of the systems involved and the severity of clinical disease;
- transmission of the condition from father to offspring does not occur.

Each cell contains at least hundreds of mitochondria, and any mtDNA mutation may affect all (homoplasmy) or only a fraction (heteroplasmy) of the total mitochondria in each cell. The phenotypic effect of any particular mutation depends on the severity of the mtDNA mutation, the proportion of mitochondria affected, and the susceptibility of various tissues to impaired mitochondrial energy metabolism. This makes the relationship between the proportion of mutant mtDNA and clinical phenotype very complex. Owing to different thresholds for susceptibility to mitochondrial energy defects, the tissues and organs involved in the clinical phenotype may vary markedly from one affected individual to another with the same mtDNA mutation, depending on the degree of heteroplasmy in each individual. Increasingly, families are being identified in which variations in the extent of the heteroplasmy in the offspring of a clinically healthy woman carrying a specific mtDNA mutation may result in some being clinically completely normal, some, for example, dying in early infancy with severe *Leigh disease*, and some being affected with clinically intermediate disease variants (mental retardation, retinitis pigmentosa, and ataxia). Figure 1.3 gives some idea of the what heteroplasmy is and how it relates to phenotype. Obtaining a family history appropriate to the recognition of this type of inheritance of a specific mtDNA mutation is particularly challenging. No clinical abnormality in a relative, no matter how apparently trivial or how different it may seem from the disease phenotype in the proband, can be dismissed.

The mutation rate for mtDNA is much higher than that for nuclear DNA,

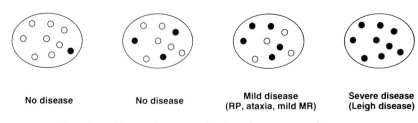

| No disease | No disease | Mild disease
(RP, ataxia, mild MR) | Severe disease
(Leigh disease) |

Fig. 1.3. The effect of heteroplasmy on the clinical expression of mtDNA mutations. The figure represents four cells, each containing nine mitochondria. Mitochondria bearing normal mtDNA are shown as open circles; those with a mtDNA mutation are shown as filled circles. As the proportion of mutant mitochondria in the cells of various tissues increases, different thresholds are reached for the production of disease-causing cell damage. While lower proportions of mutant mitochondria are well tolerated, severe disease results when the proportion is very high.

and the relative contribution of *de novo* mtDNA mutations, especially deletions, to disease is much greater than the contribution of new mutations to disease due to nuclear DNA mutations. Conditions, like *Kearns-Sayre syndrome*, which is usually the result of mtDNA deletions or duplications, are almost always sporadic, and the risk of recurrence of the condition in the family is low.

Three sources of diagnostic confusion

The commonest error in the management of inherited metabolic disorders is probably delayed or wrong diagnosis. There are three common sources of potential confusion in the diagnosis of inherited metabolic disease.

Confusion with common acquired conditions

Some inborn errors are often misdiagnosed as acquired disease, particularly some infections, intoxications, or nutritional deficiencies (Table 1.6). Failure to consider both classes of disorders simultaneously in the differential diagnosis of an acutely ill child may result in the loss of an opportunity to carry out critical diagnostic investigations, and may result in unnecessary morbidity, or even death.

Confusion caused by association with intercurrent illness

Metabolic decompensation in a child with a marginally compensated inherited metabolic disorder commonly occurs as a result of the physiological stress of intercurrent illness. Preoccupation with the intercurrent illness often delays diagnosis of the underlying genetic disorder. Owing to an impaired ability to compensate adequately for the metabolic pressures caused by intercurrent illness, particularly infection, children with inherited metabolic diseases often decom-

Table 1.6. Some common non-metabolic conditions which are often confused with inherited metabolic diseases.

Inherited metabolic 'syndrome'	Common non-metabolic disease phenocopy
Syndrome (Chapter)	*Infections*
Hepatic syndrome (5)	Hepatitis, enterovirus infection, infectious mononucleosis
Cardiomyopathy (6)	Enterovirus infection
Storage syndrome (7)	Congenital CMV infection, congenital toxoplasmosis
Encephalopathy (2)	Arbovirus infections, enterovirus infections, herpes infections (especially newborn), postinfectious encephalopathy (e.g., chicken pox)
	Intoxications
Neurologic syndrome (2)	CNS depressants, antihistaminics, anticonvulsants
Lactic acidosis (4)	Ethanol, methanol, ethylene glycol, salicylism
Hepatic syndrome (5)	Valproic acid intoxication, amiodarone reaction
Cardiac syndrome (6)	ACTH reaction (cardiomyopathy)
	Nutritional deficiencies
Lactic acidosis (4)	Thiamine deficiency
Methylmalonic acidemia (4)	Vitamin B_{12} deficiency
	Hematopoietic disorders
Storage syndrome (7)	FEL, hemoglobinopathies, lymphoma, malignant histiocytosis
Hepatic syndrome (5)	

Note: Abbreviations: CMV, cytomegalovirus; CNS, central nervous system; FEL, familial erythrophagocytic lymphohistiocytosis.

pensate when they contract relatively trivial infections. The child with intermittent MSUD (*maple syrup urine disease*) or a fatty acid oxidation defect, or the girl with OTC (*ornithine transcarbamylase*) deficiency, is often the one in the family who is described as 'sickly'. They get sicker and take longer to recover from trivial viral infections than their healthy siblings.

However, some inherited metabolic diseases significantly increase the risk of intercurrent illness. For example, recurrent, treatment-resistant, otitis media is a common problem in children of all ages with mucopolysaccharide storage diseases in which distortion of the Eustachian tube and the production of particularly tenacious mucus combine to create a favorable environment for bacterial colonization of the middle ear. The neutropenia that is a prominent feature of *glycogen storage disease* (GSD), type Ib, and some of the organic acidopathies, predisposes to pyogenic infections. Classical galactosemia predisposes infants to neonatal *Escherichia coli* sepsis by a mechanism that is not yet understood.

Confusion arising from genetic heterogeneity
Among the inherited metabolic diseases, two or more clinically similar disorders may be caused by mutations in completely different genes. This follows from the fact that the net result of a defect in any one of a number of steps in a complex metabolic process may be functionally the same. A prominent example of this is the mucopolysaccharide storage disease, Sanfilippo disease, a group of clinically indistinguishable diseases caused by defects in different enzymes involved in the breakdown of the glycosaminoglycan, heparan sulfate. This has important implications for carrier testing and for prenatal diagnosis, situations in which major decisions are made on the strength of the results of a single laboratory test. Doing the wrong test has a high probability of producing the wrong results, sometimes with tragic consequences.

Congenital malformations and inborn errors of metabolism
On the one hand, major congenital malformations, such as meningomyelocele, complex congenital heart disease, and major congenital limb deformities, are not generally considered signs of an underlying inherited metabolic disease. On the other hand, the recent discovery of a specific defect in cholesterol biosynthesis in patients with *Smith-Lemli-Opitz syndrome* has forced some modification of this view. There are some inherited metabolic conditions in which dysmorphism is so characteristic that a strong presumptive diagnosis can be made on physical examination alone. This is discussed in detail in Chapter 7.

Bibliography
Saudubray, J.M. & Ogier, H. (1990). Clinical approach to inherited metabolic disorders. In *Inborn Metabolic Diseases*, ed. J. Fernandes, J.-M. Saudubray & K. Tada, pp. 3–25. Berlin: Springer-Verlag.
Scriver, C.R., Beaudet, A.L., Sly, W.S. & Valle, D. (Editors) (1995). *The Metabolic and Molecular Bases of Inherited Disease*, 7th edn. New York: McGraw-Hill.
Schaub, J., Van Hoof, F. & Vis, H.L. (Editors) (1991). *Inborn Errors of Metabolism*. New York: Raven Press.
Thompson, M.W., McInnes, R.R. & Willard, H.F. (1991). *Genetics in Medicine*, 5th edn. Philadelphia: W.B. Saunders Company.
Vogel, F. & Motulsky, A.G. (1986). *Human Genetics*, 2nd edn. Berlin: Springer-Verlag.
Weatherall, D.J. (1991). *The New Genetics and Clinical Practice*, 3rd edn. Oxford: Oxford University Press.

2

Neurologic syndrome

Neurologic symptoms are the presenting and most prominent clinical problem associated with many inherited metabolic disorders. However, neurologic problems in general are common, especially psychomotor retardation, and deciding who to investigate, and the type of testing to be done, is often difficult. The age of onset and clinical course may provide important clues to the metabolic nature of the disorder. This is also one situation in which delineation of the extent of the pathology is often invaluable. Besides determining the range of pathology within the nervous system, it is important to establish the extent to which other organs and tissues are involved in order to make a rapid diagnosis of inherited metabolic disease.

In addition to very careful and comprehensive clinical assessment, imaging studies, electrophysiologic investigation, and histopathologic and ultrastructural information from selected biopsies help to establish the distribution and type of abnormalities within the nervous system. Some patterns of abnormalities are so typical of certain disorders that metabolic studies are required only to confirm the diagnosis. Similarly, the pattern and degree of involvement of other organs and tissues is sometimes sufficiently characteristic to suggest a specific course of metabolic investigation. On one hand, for example, the presence of retinitis pigmentosa, hepatocellular dysfunction, and renal tubular dysfunction, in a child with psychomotor retardation, muscle weakness and seizures, strongly suggests the possibility of a mitochondrial defect. On the other hand, the presence of hepatosplenomegaly without significant hepatocellular dysfunction, in a child with slowly progressive psychomotor retardation and ataxia without seizures, suggests that the pursuit of a diagnosis of a lysosomal storage disease is likely to be more productive.

Among the inherited metabolic diseases, there are five particularly common neurologic presentations:

- Chronic encephalopathy.
- Acute encephalopathy.
- Movement disorder.
- Myopathy.
- Psychiatric or behavioral abnormalities.

Chronic encephalopathy

Of all the neurologic problems that occur in patients with inherited metabolic diseases, *developmental delay* or *psychomotor retardation* is the commonest. The diagnosis of psychomotor retardation involves assessment of age appropriateness in a number of developmental spheres, including IQ in older patients, and gross motor, fine motor, socio-adaptive, and linguistic milestones in young children and infants. In young children, the Denver Developmental Screening Test is relatively easy to master and apply on a routine basis. Other screening tests are more sophisticated and require special training or access to special supplies or equipment. The periodic reports provided by teachers on the social and academic progress of a child in class provide invaluable information on development, particularly on any deterioration over a period of several months.

Psychomotor retardation is a prominent feature of many inherited metabolic diseases, but only a fraction of the mental retardation encountered in practice will turn out to be caused by inborn errors of metabolism. Who, then, should be investigated, and what type of investigation is most appropriate in each case?

Some general characteristics of the psychomotor retardation caused by inborn errors of metabolism

There are some characteristics of the cognitive disabilities caused by inherited metabolic diseases which, when present, should alert the clinician to the possibility of an underlying inborn error of metabolism.

First, *it tends to be global,* affecting all spheres of development to some extent. Although a mild developmental problem may present as delay in the development of speech, in most cases, a careful history and developmental examination show that the defect extends to the other developmental spheres. Older children with mental retardation caused by inborn errors of metabolism commonly show discrepancies in performance on tests of general intelligence, such as the Wechsler Intelligence Scale for Children (revised) (WISC-R): they often perform better on tests of verbal skills compared with motor skills. On the other hand, conditions characterized by progressive myopathy may present as developmental delay characterized by deficits limited to gross motor activities.

The nature of the underlying disability usually becomes obvious on examination.

Secondly, *severe irritability, impulsivity, aggressiveness, and hyperactivity* are also more common among infants with mental retardation caused by inborn errors of metabolism than among infants with nonmetabolic diseases. Infants with Krabbe globoid cell leukodystrophy are often implacable. Patients with *Sanfilippo disease* (MPS III) and boys with Hunter disease (MPS II) exhibit particularly disruptive behavior, which in the case of Sanfilippo disease may be the presenting complaint. Motor automatisms and stereotypic behavior are also common in these disorders. Compulsive chewing of the thumb and fingers often results in maceration of the skin and chronic paronychia. The self-mutilatory behavior of boys with *Lesch-Nyhan syndrome* (X-linked HPRT deficiency) is particularly prominent, sometimes resulting in traumatic amputation of fingers or severe laceration of the lips. Nocturnal restlessness is a common problem in both children and adults with inherited metabolic diseases affecting the brain.

Thirdly, *the psychomotor retardation is usually progressive.* There is generally a history of a period of apparently normal development, followed by loss of developmental milestones or progressive deterioration in school performance. Initially, the progression may be subtle, amounting to an apparent arrest of development during which the gap between the developmental level of the patient and normal children of the same age grows wider with time, without any obvious loss of developmental milestones. Ultimately, loss of previously acquired skills makes the progressive nature of the problem obvious.

On the one hand, earlier onset signals a more rapidly progressive course of the mental handicap. The developmental deficit in a six-year-old with a history of mild mental retardation dating from early infancy, and associated with no regression or other neurologic problems, is unlikely to be attributable to any known inherited metabolic disease. On the other hand, the progression of the intellectual deficit in late-onset *GM2 gangliosidosis* is usually very slow, tending to be obscured by the prominence of the movement disorder or psychiatric problems associated with the disease. The course of the deterioration in some inherited metabolic diseases, such as metachromatic leukodystrophy, is sigmoidal: a period of relatively slow progression is followed by rapid deterioration, which is then followed by a long period in a near-vegetative state.

It is important to distinguish primary developmental regression, occurring as a result of progression of the disease, from pseudo-regression due to environmental or other secondary effects on the nervous system (Table 2.1).

Fourthly, *the psychomotor retardation is usually associated with other objective evidence of neurologic dysfunction,* such as disorders of tone, impairment of special senses, seizures, pyramidal tract signs, evidence of extrapyramidal deficits, or

Table 2.1. *Causes of developmental pseudo-regression.*

Emotional problems, such as depression
The apparent developmental regression of emotionally disturbed infants is well-recognized. This is not a common cause of pseudo-regression in very young children, but must be considered in patients who are mature and lucid enough to be aware of their advancing disease.

Poorly controlled seizure activity
Apparent developmental regression is a common consequence of poor seizure control. The problem is particularly difficult to unravel when the seizures themselves are clinically subtle, but frequent enough to impair consciousness for significant periods of time.

Over-medication with anticonvulsants
The relationship between apparent regression and the introduction of new drugs or changes in drug dosages is usually obvious. An understanding of the usual course of the response to anticonvulsant therapy and possible drug interactions (e.g., erythromycin and carbamazepine), helps to identify this common cause of pseudo-regression.

Intercurrent systemic illness
Children with severe static brain lesions, such as cerebral palsy, often show developmental regression during intercurrent systemic illnesses. This is generally recognized to be reversible in time. However, the recovery of skills is sometimes so slow it raises the question of possible neurological regression which may prompt needless investigation. The relationship to intercurrent illness is usually obvious.

Secondary neurological problems
Secondary neurological problems arising as part of the natural history of some static brain lesions may result in the loss of some previously acquired skills. One example is the loss of mobility arising from skeletal and joint deformities caused by spasticity. A previously ambulatory child with cerebral palsy may stop walking as a result of shortening of the Achilles tendons. The resulting discrepancy between gross motor and other developmental spheres is a clue to the mechanism of the regression in these patients.

cranial nerve deficits. Moreover, the likelihood that the mental retardation is due to an inborn error of metabolism is increased if the associated neurologic deficits involve more than one part of the nervous system, such as evidence of central nervous system (CNS) disease along with signs of a peripheral neuropathy.

A general approach to the investigation of inherited metabolic causes of chronic encephalopathy is presented in Figure 2.1. It is based on the early determination of the degree of involvement of different components of the nervous system and of the extent of involvement of non-neural tissues. Those

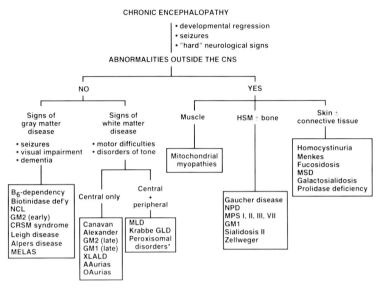

Fig. 2.1. An approach to inherited metabolic diseases with chronic encephalopathy. Abbreviations: NCL, neuronal ceroid-lipofuscinosis; CRSM, cherry-red spot-myoclonus syndrome; MELAS, mitochondrial encephalomyopathy-lactic acidosis and stroke-like episodes syndrome; XLALD, X-linked adrenoleukodystrophy; AAurias, amino acidurias; OAurias, organic acidurias; MLD, metachromatic leukodystrophy; GLD, globoid cell leukodystrophy; NPD, Niemann-Pick disease; MPS, mucopolysaccharidosis; MSD, multiple sulfatase deficiency; HSM, hepatosplenomegaly.

disorders in which metabolic acidosis is a prominent aspect of the presentation are discussed in Chapter 4. Similarly, conditions in which hepatic involvement dominates the clinical presentation are considered in Chapter 5, and conditions typically associated with unusual physical features or dysmorphism are discussed in Chapter 7.

Although this approach serves well when the clinical manifestations of disease are well established, many of the signs that are particularly characteristic of inherited metabolic diseases only emerge with observation over a period of time.

Initial investigation

A strategy for the initial investigation of young patients presenting with what might be regarded as undifferentiated chronic encephalopathy or psychomotor retardation without evidence of non-neurologic involvement is shown in Table 2.2. It includes studies to determine the extent and degree of neurologic damage,

Table 2.2. *Initial investigation of chronic encephalopathy.*

Thorough developmental assessment and neurologic examination
Brain imaging: CT or MRI scan
Electrophysiologic studies: auditory brain stem responses, visual evoked potentials,
    somatosensory evoked potentials, nerve conduction studies
Radiographs of the hands, chest, and lateral of the spine: for evidence of dysostosis
    multiplex
Plasma amino acid analysis: screening by thin-layer chromatography will meet most
    needs; quantitative amino acid analysis, if abnormalities are found
Urinary amino acid thin-layer or paper chromatography
Urinary organic acid analysis: even in the absence of overt metabolic acidosis
Plasma ammonium, preferably two hours after a normal meal of protein-containing
    food
Plasma lactate
Urinary MPS screening test
Urinary oligosaccharide screening test

Note: Abbreviation: MPS, mucopolysaccharide.

to ensure that the early stages of some treatable metabolic disorder are not missed, and to establish a baseline for monitoring the natural history of the condition.

Any metabolic abnormality would be an indication for further investigation. Primary disorders of amino acid metabolism would be unlikely to be missed through this approach. Similarly, most primary defects of organic acid metabolism would be detected, particularly those in which the psychomotor retardation is severe.

The schedule and protocol for reassessment would depend primarily on the age of the patient, the severity of the psychomotor disability, the findings at the initial investigation, and the reproductive plans of the parents. One must be alert to the emergence of new clinical signs and be prepared to depart from a protocol that might have been generated in the first place by the feeling that the problem was not the result of an inborn error of metabolism. Often the clinical signs of disease at presentation in early childhood may suggest an inherited metabolic disorder, but intensive metabolic investigation fails to demonstrate any diagnostically specific abnormality. In some cases, like *Rett syndrome*, the subsequent clinical course of the condition is sufficiently typical to indicate the diagnosis. In other situations, new information may emerge which redirects the metabolic investigation, leading to the identification of a specific primary metabolic abnormality or a new disease.

Chronic encephalopathy without non-neural involvement

Whether the signs of disease are primarily signs of gray matter or white matter involvement, or both, is a useful guide to diagnosis.

Gray matter disease

Seizures, visual failure, extrapyramidal disturbances, and dementia generally occur early in the course of gray matter diseases. Among the different variants of the same disease, onset with seizures is more common among those presenting in early infancy; late-onset variants are more likely to present with extrapyramidal movement disorders and dementia. The specific characteristics of seizures which might suggest they are the result of a primary, inherited, disorder of brain metabolism include:

• Onset early in life.
• Association with other neurologic signs, such as psychomotor retardation, disorders of tone, movement disorders, or visual impairment.
• Complex partial or myoclonic seizures.
• Resistance to conventional anticonvulsant therapy.

Intractable seizures in the newborn are considered in detail in Chapter 8. Beyond the newborn period, there are a small number of inherited metabolic diseases in which presentation as a seizure disorder is common, perhaps with little or no evidence of other problems.

One of the most difficult of this group are patients with *atypical pyridoxine-dependent seizures*. Pyridoxine-dependent seizures typically present in the newborn period (Chapter 8) as generalized tonic-clonic seizures, which are dramatically responsive to administration of large intravenous doses (100 mg) of pyridoxine (vitamin B_6). The diagnosis of atypical pyridoxine dependency is also based on the response to treatment with pyridoxine; however, the response to treatment is more variable. Rapid response to therapy seems to be the exception, and exclusion of the diagnosis may require a trial of up to 50 mg of vitamin B_6 per kilogram of body weight, given daily for at least three weeks.

Biotinidase deficiency, a form of multiple carboxylase deficiency, commonly presents between three and six months of life with failure to thrive, metabolic acidosis, a skin rash resembling seborrheic dermatitis, and alopecia, in addition to seizures (see Chapter 4). However, any of the usual features of the disorder may be absent. Some infants have been reported presenting as early as one month of age with infantile spasms. The skin rash, hair changes, and acidosis, may only develop some weeks or months later. Presumptive diagnosis is by urinary organic acid analysis, though in some infants the typical abnormalities are sometimes

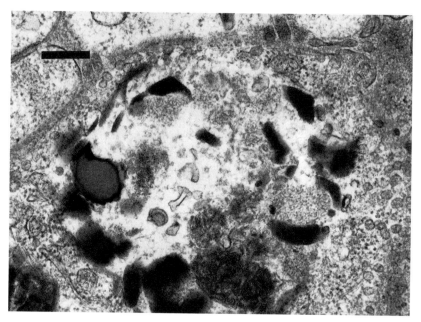

Fig. 2.2. Electron micrograph of conjunctival epithelium showing curvilinear and fingerprint inclusions in patient with neuronal ceroid-lipofuscinosis. The bar represents 1μm. (Courtesy of Dr. Venita Jay.)

absent. Confirmation of the diagnosis is by enzyme assay on as little as a few drops of blood. The response to treatment with biotin is dramatic. If the diagnosis is considered, treatment with 20 mg per day should be begun without delay while awaiting the results of laboratory studies.

Seizures may be the presenting sign of early-onset variants of *neuronal ceroid lipofuscinosis* (NCL). They are invariably a major problem in the later stages of the disease, regardless of the age of onset. Developmental delay or psychomotor regression is almost always present, usually preceeding the onset of myoclonus which may be interpreted as seizures. Visual impairment is a prominent and early feature of this disorder. It is more likely to be the presenting problem in children over the age of three years. Macular degeneration, marked attenutation of the retinal vessels, peripheral 'bone-spicule' pigment deposits, and optic atrophy are typical findings. Early extinction of the electroretinogram (ERG) is a classical feature of NCL. Electron microscopic examination of conjunctival epithelium, skin, peripheral blood leukocytes, or rectal mucosa, shows the presence of typical amorphous or membranous inclusions (Figure 2.2). Late-onset NCL tends to present with dementia or psychiatric problems.

Cherry-red spot myoclonus syndrome (sialidosis, type II) may present with seizure-like polymyoclonia in later childhood or adolescence with little or no evidence of dementia. However, vision is usually impaired, and ophthalmo-scopic examination reveals the presence of a prominent cherry-red spot in the macula. The urinary oligosaccharide pattern is usually abnormal. The diagnosis is confirmed by demonstrating deficiency of α-neuraminidase in fibroblasts.

Seizures with persistent lactic acidosis may be the first indication of an inherited metabolic disorder of mitochondrial energy metabolism, such as *pyruvate dehydrogenase* (PDH) *deficiency* or mitochondrial electron transport chain (ETC) defects. The most aggressive clinical variant of this group of disorders is *Leigh disease (subacute necrotizing encephalomyelopathy)*. It is characterized by onset of feeding difficulties and failure to thrive, usually in the first or second year of life. Seizures generally occur on a background of psychomotor retardation then regression, hypotonia, oculomotor abnormalities, episodes of recurrent apnea, ataxic breathing, and tachypnea. The course of the disease is variable. The neurologic deterioration is often punctuated by periods of partial recovery, then acute deterioration. In some infants, progression of the disease appears to arrest for periods of up to several months. There is no effective treatment for the disease, and death generally occurs within weeks to a few years after the onset of symptoms.

Persistent lactic acidosis is typical of most patients with Leigh disease, regardless of the underlying biochemical pathology. However, sometimes it is difficult to determine whether lactate accumulation is the result of a primary defect in lactic acid metabolism, or simply the normal response to uncontrolled seizure activity. In a small proportion of patients, plasma lactate levels may be normal much of the time. Measurement of cerebrospinal fluid (CSF) lactate levels is helpful in these situations. CSF lactate levels are not as likely to be spuriously elevated as plasma lactate, and they are often elevated in patients with primary disorders of lactic acid metabolism even when plasma levels are normal. Rarely, both plasma and CSF lactates are normal. Imaging studies often show destructive lesions in the basal ganglia and thalamus. Confirmation of the diagnosis requires biochemical studies on fibroblasts or skeletal muscle (see Chapter 9).

Alpers disease (progressive infantile poliodystrophy) is a clinical syndrome, similar to Leigh disease, characterized by onset in early childhood of psychomotor retardation, then regression, disturbances of tone, myoclonic or tonic-clonic seizures, ataxia, and episodic tachypnea. The principal difference is the prominence in Alpers disease of seizures and cortical blindness, a reflection of the greater involvement of the cerebral cortex. This syndrome has been reported in infants with various inborn errors of energy metabolism, particularly PDH deficiency and mitochondrial ETC defects. Persistent lactic acidosis is common, often becoming severe during intercurrent infections. The approach to diagnosis is the same as for Leigh disease.

Patients with *mitochondrial encephalomyopathy, lactic acidosis, and stroke-like episodes* (MELAS) generally present in middle-to-later childhood with a history of psychomotor delay, growth failure, headaches, vomiting, and seizures. Alternating hemiparesis and visual field defects or blindness, exercise intolerance, and muscle weakness, are also common and prominent features of the disease. During episodes of acute encephalopathy, lactate levels may rise to 10–20 mmol/L. Despite the name given to the disease, plasma lactate levels between episodes of metabolic decompensation are not always elevated. However, CSF lactate levels are generally two to three times above normal. CSF protein concentrations are also increased. Imaging studies typically show patchy cortical lucencies indicative of ischemic damage. These do not always conform to the distribution of cerebral arteries. Histochemical studies on skeletal muscle biopsies show ragged-red fibers. Biochemical studies on muscle often show deficiency of Complex I or Complexes I and IV of the mitochondrial ETC. A particularly common defect in patients with this disease is a point mutation in mitochondrial tRNA^{Leu}.

Measurement of the ratio of lactate to pyruvate (L/P) in plasma or CSF in patients with chronic progressive encephalopathy and lactic acidosis establishes whether lactate accumulation is the result of pyruvate accumulation or accumulation of NADH (see Chapter 4). If the L/P is normal, the accumulation of lactate is probably the result of a defect in pyruvate metabolism, either pyruvate carboxylase (PC) deficiency, type A, or PDH deficiency. Measurement of the enzyme activities in leukocytes or fibroblasts will confirm the diagnosis. If the L/P ratio is increased and the 3-hydroxybutyrate to acetoacetate ratio is decreased, PC deficiency, type B, should be considered, though the age of the patient and the presence of other abnormalities (hyperammonemia, and increased plasma levels of citrulline, lysine and proline) should suggest the diagnosis. Again, measurement of PC activity in leukocytes or fibroblasts confirms the diagnosis. Although mitochondrial ETC defects are sometimes identifiable from studies on cultured skin fibroblasts, confirmation of a diagnosis often requires muscle biopsy with histochemical studies, electron microscopy, and biochemical studies, on mitochondrial electron transport in mitochondria isolated fresh from the tissue (see Chapter 9).

Infants with the severe, late-infantile variants of GM2 gangliosidosis – *Tay-Sachs disease* and *Sandhoff disease* – usually present at 6–12 months of age with a history of developmental arrest, hypotonia, visual inattentiveness, markedly exaggerated startle reflex, and macrocephaly. Visual failure and seizures occur early and are difficult to control. Fundoscopic examination reveals macular cherry-red spots which, in this clinical context, are virtually pathognomonic of the disease. Although Tay-Sachs mutations are common among Ashkenazi Jews, the incidence of the disease in the Jewish community has dropped dramatically over the past 25 years as a result of carrier screening and prenatal diagnosis. In our own experience, the vast majority of affected infants seen over the past 15 years have not been Jewish. Tay-Sachs disease is caused by deficiency of β-hexosaminidase A. The diagnosis is confirmed by measurement of the enzyme in plasma, leukocytes, or fibroblasts.

Sandhoff disease is a panethnic disease which is much rarer that Tay-Sachs disease, though clinically almost indistiguishable from it. Infants with Sandhoff disease often show mild hepatomegaly, some thickening of alveolar ridges, and radiographic evidence of very mild dysostosis multiplex in addition to all the features of Tay-Sachs disease, including macrocephaly and typical macular cherry-red spots. The disease is caused by deficiency of both β-hexosaminidase A and B, which is easily demonstrated in plasma, leukocytes, or fibroblasts.

White matter disease
In diseases predominantly affecting white matter, the clinical presentation tends to be dominated by motor difficulties, including gross motor delay, weakness, and incoordination. White matter disease (leukodystrophy) is a common feature of many inherited metabolic disorders presenting with chronic encephalopathy, including many 'small molecule' diseases. Therefore, the investigation of any patient presenting with signs of leukodystrophy should routinely include analysis of plasma amino acids and urinary organic acids.

The leukodystrophy in patients with *Canavan disease* is particularly aggressive and typically associated with rapidly developing megalencephaly. Affected infants present in the first few months of life with a history of developmental arrest, irritability, hypotonia, and failure to thrive, followed by spasticity and seizures. Imaging studies show severe, diffuse white matter attentuation. The disease is caused by deficiency of aspartoacylase which is associated with accumulation of N-acetylaspartate (NAA) in the CSF, blood, and urine. Diagnosis is made by demonstrating increased NAA levels in urine, or by direct demonstration of the enzyme deficiency in fibroblasts. The incidence of this disease is high among Ashkenazi Jews in whom a single mutation (E285A) accounts for 80–85% of the mutant alleles with only two other mutations accounting for the bulk of the remainder. *Alexander disease* is a phenocopy of

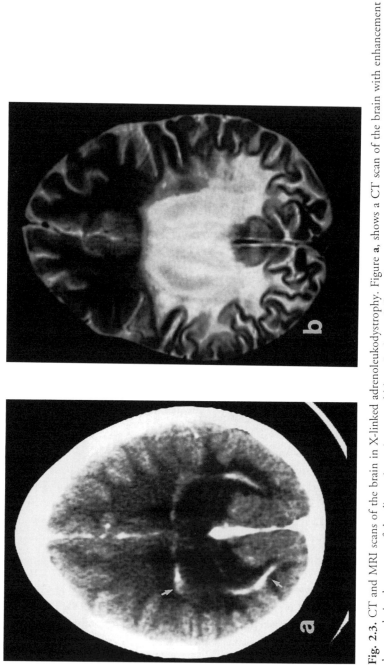

Fig. 2.3. CT and MRI scans of the brain in X-linked adrenoleukodystrophy. Figure **a**, shows a CT scan of the brain with enhancement done early in the course of the disease in a nine-year-old boy. It shows diffuse white matter attenuation in the peritrigonal area and corpus callosum. The arrows indicate the rim of active demyelination characteristic of X-linked adrenoleukodystrophy. Figure **b**, shows a T2-weighted MRI scan (TR2800/TE90) done 10 years later. It shows extensive demyelination of the peritrigonal area and corpus callosum extending into subcortical white matter with incomplete sparing of U-fibres. (Courtesy of Dr. Susan I. Blaser.)

Canavan disease with early onset of developmental arrest, hypotonia, seizures, and marked megalencephaly. Imaging studies show severe white matter disease. The biochemical basis of the disease is unknown; diagnosis is by demonstration of Rosenthal fibers in the brain at autopsy.

Boys with *X-linked adrenoleukodystrophy* (XL-ALD) generally present in middle childhood with a history of behavior problems (irritability, withdrawal, obsessiveness) or school failure, followed by the development of gait disturbances, increased muscle tone progressing to spasticity, visual failure, and deafness. Deterioration to a neuro-vegetative state occurs rapidly, though death may be delayed for some years. Some boys present with overt clinical evidence of adrenal insufficiency, such as a history of fatiguability and deep tanning of the skin. All boys with the condition show at least biochemical evidence of adrenal failure some time in the course of the disease. The CT and MRI changes are so typical that they immediately suggest the diagnosis (Figure 2.3), which is confirmed by measurement of very long-chain fatty acids in plasma.

The onset of disease in males who have inherited an XL-ALD mutation may be delayed for several years. Late-onset variants of the disease, called *adrenomyeloneuropathy* (AMN), are often clinically difficult to distinguish from progressive multiple sclerosis. Dementia is late and only very slowly progressive. However, the biochemical abnormalities are the same as in classical juvenile-onset XL-ALD. Curiously, many different clinical variants of the disease may occur in male members of the same family. This makes genetic counselling for this disorder particularly difficult.

Many patients with late-onset variants of GM2 gangliosidosis present with motor difficulties, such as ataxia, dysarthria, and dystonia, caused by generalized white matter involvement with the disease. Imaging studies show generalized brain atrophy, but posterior fossa structures are usually particularly severely affected. Unlike the common infantile-onset variants of the disease (Tay-Sachs disease and Sandhoff disease), macular cherry-red spots are not seen in patients with late-onset forms of the disease. The diagnosis is confirmed by measurement of β-hexosaminidase A and B in plasma, leukocytes, or fibroblasts.

The presence of peripheral neuropathy may not be clinically obvious, but it is an important feature of inherited disorders of myelin lipid metabolism, such as metachromatic leukodystrophy and Krabbe globoid cell leukodystrophy. *Metachromatic leukodystrophy* (MLD) is caused by deficiency of arylsulfatase A and is characterized by accumulation of the myelin lipid, sulfatide, in the brain and peripheral nerve. The clinical presentation in early onset variants of MLD is usually dominated by signs of motor difficulties, such as weakness, clumsiness, and stumbling, resembling ataxia. Nerve conduction studies show slowing, and the CSF protein concentration is characteristically elevated. Cognitive functioning is usually initially only minimally affected. The diagnosis is confirmed by measurement of arylsulfatase A in leukocytes or fibroblasts. Later in the course of the disease, and early in the course of late-onset variants of MLD, cognitive dysfunction is more prominent. Children with juvenile-onset MLD generally come to attention as a result of deteriorating school performance, though the presence of motor difficulties and some dysarthria can usually be demonstrated on careful physical examination. Long-term survival in a near-vegetative state is common in patients with MLD, irrespective of the age of onset.

Krabbe globoid cell leukodystrophy usually presents in the first few months of life with implacable irritability, marked generalized hypertonia, and developmental arrest. The course of the disease is marked by the early development of decerebrate posturing, swallowing difficulties, and blindness, progressing to early death, usually before 18 months of age. Nerve conduction is slow, and the CSF protein is elevated. The diagnosis is confirmed by the demonstration of marked deficiency of galactocerebrosidase in leukocytes or fibroblasts.

In children with peroxisomal disorders, such as *Zellweger syndrome, pseudo-Zellweger syndrome, neonatal adrenoleukodystrophy, infantile Refsum disease*, and *rhizomelic chondrodysplasia punctata*, cerebral cortical disorganization is often prominent, and seizures are a common early manifestation of the disorders. Dysmorphism, severe psychomotor retardation, sensorineural deafness, peripheral neuropathy, failure to thrive, and evidence of hepatcellular disease, may be absent or subtle compared with the seizures, particularly early in the course of the later-onset variants. These conditions are discussed in somewhat more detail in Chapter 7. Analysis of very long-chain fatty acids, pipecolic acid, and bile acid intermediates in plasma is usually sufficient to establish the diagnosis (see Chapter 9).

Chronic encephalopathy with non-neural tissue involvement

The pattern of non-neural tissue involvement in patients presenting with chronic encephalopathy is an important clinical clue to the underlying defect. Many of the diseases exhibiting significant non-neurologic involvement are caused by defects in organelle metabolism. Those in which myopathy is particularly prominent are considered in the section on 'Myopathy'.

Hepatosplenomegaly is a prominent feature of many of the lysosomal storage diseases presenting as chronic encephalopathy. In some, such as *Hurler disease* (MPS IH), *Hunter disease* (MPS II), and *Sly disease* (MPS VII) the non-neurologic manifestations of disease dominate the clinical presentation, and they are discussed in Chapter 7. Whereas, in patients with Sanfilippo disease (MPS III), the hepatosplenomegaly is rarely very impressive and the radiographic evidence of dysostosis multiplex may be very subtle. Patients with Sanfilippo disease usually present in the first few years of life with a history of developmental delay, speech retardation, and characteristically horrendous behavior problems characterized by marked impulsivity, aggressiveness, hyperactivity, stereotypic motor auto-matisms, and nocturnal restlessness. The diagnosis is often suggested on the basis of the behavior alone. The four biochemically distinct variants of Sanfilippo disease (MPS IIIA, B, C, and D) are clinically indistinguishable from each other. Urinary MPS screening tests are sometimes falsely negative. Thin-layer chromatography of urinary MPS typically shows increased excretion of heparan sulfate. The diagnosis is confirmed by analysis in fibroblasts of each of the four enzymes found deficient in different variants of the disease (see Chapter 9).

Infants with *acute neuronopathic Gaucher disease (type II)* present in the first few months of life with developmental arrest, hypertonia, neck retraction, strabismus, visual impairment, and major feeding difficulties as a result of inability to swallow. The liver and especially the spleen are typically huge, but bone changes, which are so prominent in many patients with *non-neuronopathic Gaucher disease (type I)*, do not occur. Storage cells are not seen in the peripheral circulation. However, bone marrow aspirates contain typical Gaucher cells which are indistinguishable from those seen in non-neuronopathic variants of the disease. The diagnosis is confirmed by demonstrating deficiency of lysosomal β-glucosidase (or glucocerebrosidase) in leukocytes or fibroblasts. Most infants with acute neuronopathic Gaucher disease carry at least one L444P mutation. This is a rapidly progressive disease, generally ending in death before age two years.

Children with *subacute neuronopathic Gaucher disease (type III)* usually present in early childhood with aggressive visceral disease. On the one hand, there may not be any obvious clinical evidence of neurologic involvement for some years. On the other hand, affected patients typically show an unsual oculomotor abnormality, characterized by vertically looping movements of the eyes on sacchadic lateral gaze, sometimes long before the development of other neurological abnormalities. Superficially, the disease resembles a very severe form of non-neuronopathic Gaucher disease. In fact, some patients die of hepatic failure before they develop significant neurologic problems. Biochemically, patients with this disease are indistinguishable from patients with severe non-neuronopathic Gaucher disease (see Chapter 7).

Infants with *Niemann-Pick disease* (NPD), especially type A, also present in the first few months of life with typically massive enlargement of the liver and spleen causing marked protuberance of the abdomen. However, serious neurologic involvement with the disease occurs later and is more slowly progressive than in Gaucher disease. Feeding problems commonly cause severe failure to thrive, and pulmonary involvement often causes chronic respiratory problems. Liver function tests may be mildly abnormal. Skeletal radiographs are usually normal. However, radiographs of the chest commonly show diffuse reticular infiltrations of the lungs. Bone marrow smears usually show the presence of foamy storage histiocytes which are typical but not specific for the disease. The disease is caused by deficiency of lysosomal acid sphingomyelinase. The diagnosis of the disease is confirmed by measuring the enzyme in leukocytes or fibroblasts.

NPD, type C (NPD-C), may present in infancy or early childhood as hepatic syndrome (see Chapter 5), or later in childhood as a progressive neurodegenerative condition with little evidence of visceral involvement. Presentation as neurologic disease is usually in early to middle childhood with a progressive gait disturbance, dysarthria, emotional lability, and intellectual regression. The liver and spleen are usually enlarged, and liver function tests are often mildly abnormal. One of the characteristic features of the condition is early-onset supranuclear gaze palsy, manifested as impaired vertical sacchadic eye movements. Bone marrow aspirates show the presence of foamy histiocytes and 'sea-blue' histiocytes. The basic biochemical defect in NPD-C is not known. However, cholesterol esterification is typically markedly impaired in cultured skin fibroblasts. Fibroblasts also show strong fibrillin staining as a result of cholesterol accumulation in the cells. Confirming the diagnosis of NPD-C by laboratory studies is often difficult because the diagnostic abnormality is almost certainly a secondary manifestation of the primary metabolic defect.

GM1 gangliosidosis and *sialidosis*, along with other glycoproteinoses, are reviewed in Chapter 7. Both conditions may present in early infancy with severe, rapidly progressive, neurovisceral storage disease, associated with dysmorphic facial features resembling Hurler disease but without corneal clouding, often with cherry-red macular spots, and radiographic evidence of bone involvement. Patients with later-onset variants usually have only mild non-neurologic abnormalities. As a rule, they present with gait disturbances and dysarthria. Spasticity, seizures, and psychomotor regression follow. Analysis of urinary oligosaccharides is abnormal in both conditions. Definitive diagnosis requires demonstration of deficiency of β-galactosidase in plasma, leukocytes, or fibroblasts in the case of GM1 gangliosidosis. Confirmation of the diagnosis of sialidosis requires demonstration of α-neuraminidase deficiency in fibroblasts.

Fucosidosis and *mannosidosis* commonly present as chronic encephalopathy with developmental delay. Although both, especially fucosidosis, are associated

ACUTE ENCEPHALOPATHY

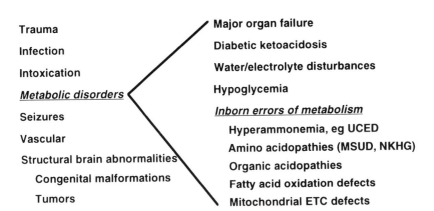

Trauma

Infection

Intoxication

Metabolic disorders

Seizures

Vascular

Structural brain abnormalities

Congenital malformations

Tumors

Major organ failure

Diabetic ketoacidosis

Water/electrolyte disturbances

Hypoglycemia

Inborn errors of metabolism

Hyperammonemia, eg UCED

Amino acidopathies (MSUD, NKHG)

Organic acidopathies

Fatty acid oxidation defects

Mitochondrial ETC defects

Fig. 2.4. Summary of major causes of acute encephalopathy.
Abbreviations: UCED, urea cycle enzyme defects; MSUD, maple syrup urine
disease; NKHG, nonketotic hyperglycinemia; ETC, electron transport chain.

with the development of 'storage facies' as they grow older, psychomotor
retardation is often the only clinical complaint at initial presentation. Radiographic evidence of mild dysostosis multiplex is usually present, though often
overlooked. Vacuolated mononuclear cells are often found in peripheral blood
smears. Patients with mannosidosis characteristically develop sensorineural
hearing loss early in the course of their disease. Angiokeratoma, indistinguishable
from those seen in patients with Fabry disease, are a typical feature of fucosidosis.

The non-neurologic features of *homocystinuria* and *Menkes disease* clearly set
them apart from other inherited metabolic diseases in which chronic encephalopathy is a prominent aspect of the clinical presentation. They are discussed in
Chapter 7.

Acute encephalopathy

Acute encephalopathy, regardless of the cause, is a medical emergency. In
addition to being a common manifestation of a variety of acquired medical or
surgical conditions, it is a presenting feature of a number of inherited metabolic
diseases, particularly in young children (Figure 2.4). Deterioration of consciousness occurring as a result of inherited metabolic disease:

• often occurs with little warning in a previously healthy infant or child;
• may be missed because the early signs may be mistaken as a behavior disorder;

Table 2.3. *Causes of metabolic acute encephalopathy to be considered at various ages.*

Condition	Age Newborn	Early childhood	Later childhood
Urea cycle defects	++++	+ (girls with OTC)	(+)
NKHG	++++	0	0
Organic acidopathies	++++	+	(+)
MSUD	++++	++	++
FAOD	+	++++	?
Reye syndrome	0	++	+++
Drug ingestion	+ (maternal)	+++	+++

Note: Abbreviations: UCED, urea cycle enzyme defects; NKHG, nonketotic hyperglycinemia; MSUD, maple syrup urine disease; FAOD, fatty acid oxidation defects; OTC, ornithine transcarbamylase deficiency.

- often progresses rapidly, may fluctuate markedly;
- usually shows no focal neurologic deficits.

The earliest signs of encephalopathy may be no more obvious than excessive drowsiness, unusual behavior, or some unsteadiness of gait. Acute or intermittent ataxia is a common sign of acute encephalopathy in older children with inborn errors of metabolism. A history of recurrent attacks of unsteadiness of gait or ataxia, especially when associated with vomiting or deterioration of consciousness, should be considered a strong indication for investigation of a possible inherited metabolic disease.

The progression to stupor and coma is often irregular, with periods of apparent lucidity alternating with periods of obtundation. Failure to recognize the inherent instability of the situation, and to monitor clinical neurologic vital signs closely, may end in disaster. The likely causes of acute metabolic encephalopathy are age-dependent (Table 2.3).

Initial investigation

Because of the importance of identifying treatable inherited metabolic diseases early, initial investigation of any patient presenting stuporous or obtunded must not be delayed (Table 2.4).

Table 2.4. *Initial investigation of acute encephalopathy.*

Blood gases and electrolytes (calculate anion gap), blood glucose
Urinalysis, including tests for ketones and reducing substances
Liver function tests
Blood ammonia
Plasma lactate
Urinary organic acids (15 ml urine, no preservative)
Plasma amino acid analysis, quantitative
Plasma carnitine and acylcarnitines

Table 2.5. *Differential diagnosis of inherited metabolic diseases presenting as acute encephalopathy.*

	UCED	MSUD	OAuria	FAOD	ETC defects
Metabolic acidosis	0	±	+++	±	++
Plasma glucose	N	N or ↓	↓↓	↓↓↓	N
Urinary ketones	N	↑↑	↑↑	0	0
Plasma ammonium	↑↑↑	N	↑↑	↑	N
Plasma lactate	N	N	↑	±	↑↑↑
Liver function	± N	N	N	↑↑	N
Plasma carnitine	N	N	↓↓↓	↓↓	N
Plasma amino acids	Abnormal	↑ BCAA	↑ glycine	±	↑ alanine
Urinary organic acids	N	Abnormal	Abnormal	Abnormal	N

Note: Abbreviations: UCED, urea cycle enzyme defect; MSUD, maple syrup urine disease; OAuria, organic aciduria; FAOD, fatty acid oxidation defect; ETC, mitochondrial electron transport chain; BCAA, branched-chain amino acids; ↑, elevated; ↓ decreased; +, present; ±, variably present; N, normal; 0, not present.

A summary of the results of initial laboratory studies in various inborn errors of metabolism presenting as acute encephalopathy is shown in Table 2.5.

Hyperammonemia

The plasma or blood ammonium should be measured *immediately* in any child presenting with acute or subacute encephalopathy of obscure etiology. However, the interpretation of the results requires additional information. Plasma ammonium levels are often elevated in patients with severe hepatocellular dysfunction, regardless of the cause, including viral infections, intoxications, or some inborn errors of metabolism. Inherited metabolic diseases presenting with hyperammonemia due to liver failure are discussed in Chapter 5. Apart from

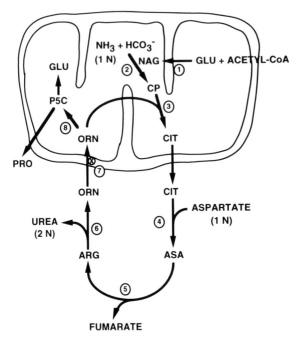

Fig. 2.5. Summary of normal ammonium metabolism

The various enzymes or transport systems involved are: **1**, N-acetylglutamate synthetase (NAGS); **2**, carbamylphosphate synthetase I (CPS I); **3**, ornithine transcarbamylase (OTC); **4**, argininosuccinic acid synthetase (ASA synthetase); **5**, argininosuccinic acid lyase (ASA lyase); **6**, arginase; **7**, mitochondrial ornithine transport system; **8**, ornithine aminotransferase. Other abbreviations: GLU, glutamate; CIT, citrulline; ARG, arginine; ORN, ornithine; P5C, Δ^1-pyrroline-5-carboxylic acid; PRO, proline. The figure shows how one of the waste nitrogens excreted as urea is derived from ammonia (NH_3); the other comes from the amino acid, aspartate.

marked elevation of plasma ammonium levels, liver function tests in patients with primary disorders of urea biosynthesis are usually near normal. Ornithine transcarbamylase (OTC) deficiency is an exception to this generalization. Transaminases in patients with the disease are often mildly to moderately elevated, but the hyperammonemia is generally much more severe than can be explained by the degree of hepatocellular dysfunction, as reflected by the transaminases and other tests of liver cell damage.

The investigation and diagnosis of possible urea cycle enzyme defects (UCED) is facilitated by reference to a simplified diagram showing the main elements of ammonium metabolism (Figure 2.5).

The key features of the metabolism of waste nitrogen are:

- The process is divided between two sets of reactions, one set in the cytosol, the other inside mitochondria.
- The first reaction, the carbamylphosphate synthase I (CPS I)-catalyzed condensation of ammonium with bicarbonate to form carbamylphosphate, requires the presence of *N*-acetylglutamate (NAG), an obligatory effector, not a substrate, for the reaction.
- One of the two waste nitrogens which become part of urea is derived from the non-essential amino acid, aspartate. Aspartate is produced by transamination of oxaloacetate in a reaction catalyzed by liver and muscle aspartate aminotransferase (AST).
- The entire process is highly dependent on an adequate supply of intra-mitochondrial ornithine.

Ornithine is a five-carbon amino acid analogue of the essential amino acid, lysine. It is formed from arginine by a reaction catalyzed by arginase. The concentration of the amino acid is directly related to the availability and metabolism of arginine. Ornithine is not incorporated into body protein. Transport into mitochondria is facilitated by a specific carrier system. Ornithine is a precursor in the biosynthesis of spermine and putrescine, as well as the amino acids, glutamate and proline.

Intramitochondrial ornithine condenses with carbamylphosphate in a reaction catalysed by OTC, which is coded by a gene on the short arm of the X chromosome. The product, citrulline, diffuses out of the mitochondrion where it condenses with aspartate to form argininosuccinic acid (ASA) in a reaction catalyzed by ASA synthetase. ASA is cleaved to produce arginine and fumarate in a reaction catalyzed by ASA lyase. The renal clearance of ASA is extremely high.

A widely used algorithmic approach to the differential diagnosis of hyperammonemic encephalopathy is presented in Figure 2.6. The presence of moderate to severe metabolic acidosis indicates that the hyperammonemia is a manifestation of an inherited disturbance of organic acid metabolism which is discussed in Chapter 4.

Urea cycle enzyme defects presenting as acute hyperammonemic encephalopathy, whether in early infancy or later in childhood, are clinically indistinguishable from each other. The most important diagnostic information, after ammonium determination, liver function tests, and analysis of blood gases and plasma glucose and electrolytes, is *quantitative* analysis of plasma amino acids. The reliance on semi-quantitative or screening tests to measure amino acid levels

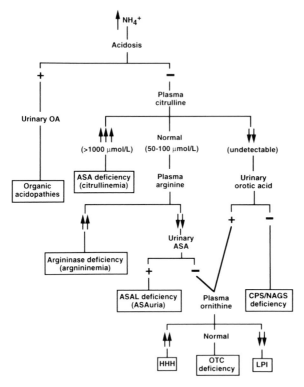

Fig. 2.6. An approach to the diagnosis of hyperammonemia in older children. Abbreviations: OA, organic acids; ASAS deficiency, argininosuccinic acid synthetase deficiency; ASAL deficiency, argininosuccinic acid lyase deficiency; CPS/NAGS, carbamylphosphate synthetase I or N-acetylglutamate synthetase; HHH, hyperammonemia-hyperornithinemia-homocitrullinemia syndrome; OTC deficiency, ornithine transcarbamylase deficiency; LPI, lysinuric protein intolerance.

is a common error in the investigation of inherited metabolic diseases. In the investigation of a patient with hyperammonemia, these are particularly inappropriate. Low concentrations of certain amino acids are as important as excesses in the differential diagnosis of hyperammonemia, and subnormal amino acid levels cannot be detected by any of the qualitative or semi-quantitative amino acid screening tests (see Chapter 9). The analytical chemist should be alerted to the need to identify low levels of amino acids as well as excesses.

The concentration of citrulline is central to the interpretation of the results of amino acid analyses. If the citrulline concentration is markedly elevated, the child has citrullinemia as a result of ASA synthetase deficiency. Citrulline levels that are extremely low suggest the presence of a defect in citrulline biosynthesis, the result of deficiency of OTC, CPS I, or NAG synthetase (NAGS).

OTC deficiency is transmitted as an X-linked recessive condition. Affected boys usually present in the newborn period with very severe, usually life-threatening, hyperammonemia. Symptomatic carrier girls generally present later in childhood with an antecedent history of feeding problems, failure to thrive, intermittent ataxia, or intermittent encephalopathy. Unfortunately, the diagnosis in the majority of symptomatic girls is often missed until the patients present with acute encephalopathy, commonly resulting in irreparable brain damage. Deficiency of OTC causes accumulation of carbamylphosphate and ammonium; diffusion of the excess carbamylphosphate into the cytosol results in over-production of pyrimidines and the pyrimidine intermediates – orotic acid and orotidine. OTC is differentiated from CPS I and NAGS deficiencies by the demonstration of increased concentrations of orotic acid and orotidine in the urine, occurring as a secondary consequence of carbamylphosphate accumulation.

Citrulline levels that are normal or only moderately elevated are generally an indication of *argininosuccinic aciduria*, the result of argininosuccinic acid lyase deficiency, or *argininemia*, caused by arginase deficiency. However, argininemia almost never presents as an acute encephalopathy. Instead, patients with this disorder tend to have only mild to moderate elevations of plasma ammonium, and they present clinically later in infancy and early childhood with 'cerebral palsy'. The elevation of plasma arginine is generally sufficiently specific to make the diagnosis.

Argininosuccinic aciduria is characterized by subnormal arginine levels in plasma and the presence of markedly increased amounts of the amino acid, argininosuccinate, in plasma and urine. The renal clearance of this amino acid is very high, and the concentrations in urine are generally very high compared with the levels in plasma. However, the demonstration of the presence of increased concentrations of argininosuccinate in plasma require no more analysis than has already been done for the normal quantitative analysis of plasma amino acids.

Lysinuric protein intolerance (LPI) may also present in later infancy or early childhood as hyperammonemic encephalopathy. This is a very protean metabolic disorder which may present as growth retardation and hepatomegaly, hematologic abnormalities, pulmonary disease, or renal disease. It is caused by a generalized hereditary defect in dibasic amino acid transport. Plasma arginine, ornithine, and lysine levels are typically markedly subnormal. At the same time, quantitative analysis of urinary amino acids shows marked increases in the excretion of the same compounds. Intracellular ornithine deficiency causes accumulation of carbamylphosphate and ammonium resulting in increased urinary orotic acid and orotidine excretion.

Hyperammonemia-hyperornithinemia-homocitrullinemia syndrome (HHH syndrome) is another disorder of ammonium metabolism caused by a defect in amino acid transport. In this case, the transport of ornithine into mitochondria is defective, resulting in intramitochondrial ornithine deficiency. Paradoxically, plasma ornithine levels are markedly elevated in this condition. However, intramitochondrial ornithine deficiency causes accumulation of carbamylphosphate and ammonium, and in the same manner as in LPI, this causes carbamylphosphate accumulation resulting in increased urinary orotic acid and orotidine concentrations.

Leucine encephalopathy (maple syrup urine disease – MSUD)

This usually presents in the newborn period as an acute encephalopathy, initially without metabolic acidosis (Chapter 8). Milder variants of the disease may present at any age in childhood. Acute encephalopathy without hyperammonemia or significant metabolic acidosis, on a background of chronic failure to thrive and mild to moderate psychomotor retardation, is typical of MSUD. Decompensation is usually heralded by drowsiness, anorexia, and vomiting. The odor widely described as resembling the aroma of maple syrup is more like the smell of burnt sugar. The urine typically tests positive for ketones. Testing the urine for the presence of α-ketoacids by addition of DNPH (dinitrophenylhydrazine) reagent produces a strongly positive reaction. Plasma ammonium levels are characteristically normal. The course of subsequent deterioration is often highly irregular with periods of lucidity alternating with stupor, progressing to coma. Signs of intracranial hypertension (posturing, dilated and sluggish pupils, periodic breathing) are an indication that the situation is grave and the chances of recovery, even with aggressive treatment, are seriously compromised. Quantitative analysis of plasma amino acids is the most rapid and reliable method to confirm the diagnosis, and it should be done without delay. Marked elevations of leucine, isoleucine, and valine, and the presence of alloisoleucine, are diagnostic of MSUD. Modest increases in branched-chain amino acids are common in children during short-term starvation and should not be confused with mild variants of MSUD.

Analysis of urinary organic acids as oxime derivatives shows the presence of a number of branched-chain α-ketoacids. However, this generally takes longer than plasma amino acid analysis and does not add much to the diagnosis of MSUD.

Reye-like acute encephalopathy (fatty acid oxidation defects)

Acute encephalopathy resembling Reye syndrome is a common presenting feature of the primary inherited disorders of fatty acid oxidation. The commonest of these is *medium-chain acyl-CoA dehydrogenase* (MCAD) *deficiency*. Affected children are usually competely well until they present, usually in the first year or two of life, with what may appear initially to be nothing more than 'stomach flu', with anorexia, vomiting, drowsiness, and lethargy. The fact that metabolic decompensation is usually precipitated by intercurrent illness, generally associated with poor feeding, often obscures the nature of the underlying metabolic disorder. Drowsiness and lethargy progress rapidly to stupor and coma, hepatomegaly with evidence of hepatocellular dysfunction, hypotonia, hypoketotic hypoglycemia (see Chapter 5), and mild to moderate hyperammonemia. Although the disease is often clinically indistinguishable from Reye syndrome, onset in the first two years of life, a positive family history, and recurrence of acute metabolic decompensation during trivial intercurrent illnesses or fasting, are features peculiar to MCAD deficiency and other fatty acid oxidation defects.

Acute encephalopathy can also occur in the absence of hypoglycemia or significant hepatocellular dysfunction, suggesting that accumulation of fatty acid oxidation intermediates plays some role in its pathogenesis. Sudden unexpected death is tragically common in infants with unrecognized MCAD deficiency, perhaps as a result of cardiac arrhythmias caused by accumulated fatty acid oxidation intermediates. Successful management of this condition rests on a high index of suspicion coupled with early treatment with glucose while awaiting the results of definitive laboratory tests.

Analysis of urinary organic acids during acute metabolic decompensation characteristically shows the presence of large amounts of C-6 to C-10 dicarboxylic acids (adipic, suberic, and sebacic acids), the (ω-1)-hydroxy derivatives of hexanoic and octanoic acids, but little or no ketones (see Chapter 5). Urinary organic acid analysis when the child is clinically well may be completely normal. However, analysis of acylcarnitines and acylglycines generally shows the presence of octanoylcarnitine, and hexanoylglycine and phenylpropionylglycine, respectively, in urine. Analysis of organic acids in plasma or dried blood spots by gas chromatography-mass spectrometry (GC-MS) shows accumulation of *cis*-4-decenoic acid which is virtually pathognomonic of MCAD deficiency.

MCAD deficiency is an inherited metabolic disorder in which specific mutation analysis is particularly useful for making a diagnosis: one mutation,

Table 2.6. *Organic acid abnormalities in the hereditary fatty acid oxidation defects.*

MCAD deficiency	SCAD deficiency	LCAD deficiency	LCHAD deficiency	ETF/ETF-DH deficiency
5-hydroxyhexanoate	**ethylmalonate**	adipate	adipate	3-hydroxybutyrate
adipate	**methylsuccinate**	suberate	3-hydroxyadipate	**glutarate**
suberate		octenedioic	suberate	**ethylmalonate**
octenedioic	**butyrylglycine**	decenedioate	octenedioate	**methylsuccinate**
7-hydroxyoctanoate		**dodecanedioate**	**3-hydroxysuberate**	
sebacate		**tetradecanedioate**	sebacate	*n*-butyrylglycine
decenedioate			decenedioate	isobutyrylglycine
3-hydroxysebacate			**3-hydroxysebacate**	2-methylbutyrylglycine
			dodecanedioate	**isovalerylglycine**
hexanoylglycine			**3-hydroxydodecanedioate**	**hexanoylglycine**
suberylglycine			**3-hydroxydodecenedioate**	
phenylpropionylglycine			**3-hydroxytetradecanedioate**	
			3-hydroxytetradecenedioate	
octanoylcarnitine				

Note: Abbreviations: MCAD, medium-chain acyl-CoA dehydrogenase; SCAD, short-chain acyl-CoA dehydrogenase; LCAD, long-chain acyl-CoA dehydrogenase; LCHAD, long-chain 3-hydroxyacyl-CoA dehydrogenase; ETF/ETF-DH, electron transport flavoprotein/electron transport flavoprotein dehydrogenase.
Bold type indicates the presence of the compound which is particularly characteristic of the disease.

K329E, accounts for over 90% of all MCAD mutant alleles discovered to date. Testing for the presence of this mutation provides helpful confirmatory evidence for this deficiency.

Other inborn errors of fatty acid oxidation are rare compared with MCAD deficiency. *Systemic carnitine deficiency* and *long-chain acyl-CoA dehydrogenase* (LCAD) *deficiency* may present with a Reye-like encephalopathy, but the evidence of skeletal muscle involvement is usually more obvious, and cardiomyopathy, which is virtually never seen in MCAD deficiency, is generally prominent. Similarly, *short-chain acyl-CoA dehydrogenase* (SCAD) *deficiency* is very rare, and usually presents as encephalopathy with metabolic acidosis in the newborn period (see Chapter 8). Rarely, *carnitine palmitoyltransferase II* (CPT II) *deficiency*, which is usually associated with a myopathy presenting in later childhood, may present in infancy with recurrent Reye-like acute encephalopathy clinically indistinguishable from MCAD deficiency. A summary of the urinary organic acid abnormalities in these conditions is shown in Table 2.6

Acute encephalopathy with metabolic acidosis

The inherited organic acidopathies commonly present as acute encephalopathy, though the presence of severe metabolic acidosis is usually recognized early in the management of the problem. Detailed treatment of this particular group of disorders is presented in Chapter 4 and Chapter 8.

Hypoglycemia

Although conditions like glycogen storage disease, type I (GSD I), often present in infancy with alteration of consciousness, sometimes progressing rapidly to coma and to seizures, the presence of hypoglycemia generally directs the investigation (see Chapter 5).

Movement disorder

Extrapyramidal movement disorders in patients with inborn errors of metabolism are almost always associated with neurologic signs referable to other parts of the nervous system (Table 2.7). Unsteadiness of gait, particularly in children, which may be a manifestation of immaturity or muscle weakness, is a particularly common finding in inherited metabolic diseases.

Progressive ataxia may be the presenting symptom in many of the late-onset variants of organelle diseases. Differentiation from nonmetabolic hereditary ataxias is usually possible on the basis of the presence of other neurologic signs, such as psychomotor retardation or regression, spasticity, or peripheral neuropathy, and evidence of non-neurologic involvement with the disease.

Table 2.7. *Inherited metabolic diseases in which extrapyramidal movement disorders are prominent.*

Disease	Other clinical features	Diagnosis
Progressive ataxia		
L-2-Hydroxyglutaric aciduria	Psychomotor retardation, choreoathetosis ± seizures	Marked increase in levels of L-2-hyroxyglutaric acid in the urine
Abetalipoproteinemia	Steatorrhea, anemia, acanthocytosis, psychomotor retardation, retinitis pigmentosa	Marked deficiency of apolipoprotein B in plasma
Infantile NCL (Santavuori-Hagberg syndrome)	Psychomotor retardation, myoclonic seizures, blindness, early flattening of the EEG	Typical lysosomal inclusions seen on electron microscopic examination of skin, leukocytes, or conjunctival epithelium
Mitochondrial ETC defects (e.g. KSS, MERRF)	Lactic acidosis, small stature, retinal degeneration, psychomotor retardation, seizures, sensorineural deafness	Defects in mitochondrial ETC in fibroblasts or skeletal muscle; mitochondrial mutation analysis
Late-onset galactosialidosis	Myoclonus, seizures, corneal clouding, cherry-red spots, mental retardation	Deficiency of β-galactosidase and α-neuraminidase in fibroblasts
Late-onset GM2 gangliosidosis	Muscle wasting, dysarthria, exaggerated deep tendon reflexes, psychosis	Deficiency of β-hexosaminidase in serum, leukocytes, or fibroblasts.
Late-onset MLD	Muscle wasting, dysarthria, peripheral neuropathy	Deficiency of arylsulfatase A in leukocytes or fibroblasts
Late-onset Krabbe GLD	Spasticity, visual failure	Deficiency of galactocerebrosidase in leukocytes or fibroblasts
Refsum disease	Retinitis pigmentosa, peripheral neuropathy, sensorineural deafness, cataracts, ichthyosis	Elevated phytanic acid levels in plasma; defect in phytanic acid oxidation in fibroblasts
Niemann-Pick disease, type C	Hepatosplenomegaly, supranuclear vertical gaze palsy, sea-blue histiocytes in bone marrow	Defect in cholesterol esterification in fibroblasts
Hartnup disease	Pellagra-like skin rash	Massive neutral, monoaminomonocarboxylic aminoaciduria
Cerebrotendinous xanthomatosis	Dementia, cataracts, spasticity, tendinous xanthomas, dysarthria	Increased cholestanol levels in plasma

Intermittent ataxia

Disease	Clinical features	Biochemical findings
UCED (e.g., OTC deficiency, CPS I deficiency, ASAuria, etc.)	Encephalopathy, dietary protein intolerance, hyperammonemia	Plasma amino acid abnormalities and deficiency of specific urea cycle enzymes
PDH deficiency (mild)	Lactic acidosis	Deficiency of PDH in leukocytes and fibroblasts
Organic acidopathies (e.g., MMA, PA, IVA)	Metabolic acidosis, hyperammonemia	Marked excretion of organic acid intermediates in the urine

Dystonia/choreoathetosis

Disease	Clinical features	Biochemical findings
Glutaric aciduria, type I	Psychomotor retardation, episodes of acute encephalopathy with metabolic acidosis	Marked increase in excretion of glutaric acid in the urine; deficiency of glutaryl-CoA dehydrogenase in fibroblasts
Lesch-Nyhan disease	Psychomotor retardation, self-mutilatory behaviour	Increased uric acid levels in plasma and urine; HPRT deficiency in leukocytes and fibroblasts
TPI deficiency	Chronic hemolytic anemia, susceptibility to infection, cardiomyopathy, death in early childhood	Deficiency of TPI in erythrocytes
4-Hydroxybutyric aciduria	Psychomotor retardation, oculomotor abnormalities, abnormalities of muscle tone, choreoathetosis	Massive excretion of 4-hydroxybutyric acid in urine, decreasing with age
Segawa syndrome	Dystonia of extremities worst in the morning improving during the day, normal intellect	Dramatic response to treatment with dopa

Parkinsonism

Disease	Clinical features	Biochemical findings
Wilson disease	Dementia, psychiatric problems, hepatocellular dysfunction (Chapter 5), Kayser-Fleischer rings	Marked decrease of plasma ceruloplasmin and copper levels and increased urinary excretion of copper

Note: Abbreviations: MLD, metachromatic leukodystrophy; ETC, electron transport chain; KSS, Kearns-Sayre syndrome; MERRF, myoclonic epilepsy and ragged-red fiber disease; NCL, neuronal ceroid lipofuscinosis; UCED, urea cycle enzyme defects; CPS I, carbamylphosphate synthetase I; ASAuria, argininosuccinic aciduria; PDH, pyruvate dehydrogenase; MMA, methylmalonic acidemia; PA, propionic acidemia; IVA, isovaleric acidemia; HPRT, hypoxanthine phosphoribosyltransferase; TPI, triose phosphate isomerase; GLD, globoid cell leukodystrophy.

Intermittent ataxia is a common manifestation of metabolic decompensation in patients with 'small molecule' disorders, such as urea cycle enzyme defects, organic acidopathies, and the mild or intermittent variants of MSUD. It may be the only clinical manifestation of mild PDH deficiency. In any child presenting with a history of recurrent episodes of ataxia, separated by periods free of neurologic abnormalities, the possibility of an inherited metabolic disease should be considered.

Choreoathetosis is a prominent feature of Lesch-Nyhan syndrome, caused by X-linked hypoxanthine phosphoribosyltransferase (HPRT) deficiency. Many, though not all, patients with the disease show psychomotor retardation. Self-mutilation, another feature of the condition in many affected boys, may not be present. The diagnosis is suggested by finding increased uric acid levels in blood and urine, and it is confirmed by specific enzyme assay on leukocytes or fibroblasts. Choreoathetosis and dystonia are characteristic of glutaric aciduria, type I. This disorder, caused by deficiency of glutaryl-CoA dehydrogenase, is characterized by the acute onset in early infancy of intermittent episodes of encephalopathy with ketoacidosis, hypotonia, seizures, posturing (arching, grimacing, tongue-thrusting, rigidity), and evidence of hepatocellular dysfunction. Recovery is usually incomplete, with the extrapyramidal movement disorder tending to persist. The urine usually contains large amounts of glutaric acid and smaller amounts of 3-hydroxyglutaric acid, though sometimes the organic acid pattern is not abnormal.

Parkinsonism, dystonia, and cerebellar dysfunction are prominent symptoms in many patients with *Wilson disease*. Most patients with the disease come to medical attention in later childhood with evidence of severe hepatocellular dysfunction (see Chapter 5). However, many present somewhat later, in adolescence or early adulthood, with neuropsychiatric problems, usually dominated by extrapyramidal or cerebellar dysfunction, or psychiatric disturbances. Cerebellar ataxia is often associated with tremors, titubation, dysmetria, and scanning speech. In other patients, symptoms of extrapyramidal disease dominate, with dystonia, cog-wheel rigidity, facial grimacing, drooling, dysphagia, and stereotypic gestures. In spite of profound disturbances of motor function, intelligence usually remains normal. Psychiatric problems are often prominent. They may even be the first indication of disease (see Table 2.13).

Myopathy

Inherited metabolic disorders presenting as myopathy are commonly the result of defects in energy metabolism. These can be divided into four categories on the basis of the clinical characteristics of the muscle disease and associated findings:

- Progressive muscle weakness.
- Exercise intolerance with cramps and myoglobinuria (myophosphorylase deficiency phenotype).
- Exercise intolerance with cramps and myoglobinuria (CPT II deficiency phenotype).
- Myopathy as a manifestation of multisystem disease (mitochondrial myopathies).

Progressive muscle weakness

One of the most striking examples of inherited metabolic diseases presenting with progressive myopathy is *Pompe disease* (GSD II), caused by deficiency of the lysosomal enzyme, α-glucosidase (acid maltase). It is characterized by the onset, at three to five months, of rapidly progressive weakness and hypotonia. Affected infants are remarkable for the marked paucity of spontaneous movement and their frog-leg posture, but who have normal social interaction. The face is myopathic, and the tongue is characteristically enlarged; however, extraocular movements are spared. Despite marked muscle weakness and hypotonia, muscle bulk is initially not significantly decreased, and the muscles have a peculiar woody texture on palpation. Deep tendon reflexes, which may initially be preserved, are soon lost. The liver is not significantly enlarged unless the infant is in heart failure. Cardiac muscle involvement is prominent and severe (see Chapter 6). The course of the disease is relentlessly progressive, culminating in death within a few months. The excess glycogen in the muscles of infants with Pompe disease accumulates in lysosomes, and lysosomal glycogen contributes next to nothing to meeting the energy needs of the tissue. Why the muscle weakness in the disease is so severe is not understood.

In late-onset variants of *acid maltase deficiency*, the onset of the myopathy is more insidious and the progression more gradual. Muscle biopsy typically shows the presence of large accumulations of intra-lysosomal glycogen.

Progressive skeletal myopathy, sometimes involving the heart, may be a major problem in patients with *glycogen storage disease, type III* (GSD III). This disease is caused by deficiency of glycogen debrancher enzyme, usually in liver and muscle, but sometimes only in liver. While the consequences of liver involvement usually improve with age (see Chapter 5), the myopathy gradually becomes worse, often only becoming clinically significant after age 20 or 30 years. The creatine phosphokinase (CPK) is often, though not always, elevated in patients with muscle involvement. The mechanism of the myopathy in GSD III is uncertain. Some feel that it is the result of local glycogen accumulation; others think, on the basis of apparent improvement using high protein dietary

Table 2.8. *Protocol for the ischemic forearm exercise test.*

1. An intravenous is established in one arm with an ample needle in the antecubital vein kept open with a slow infusion of 0.9% NaCl.
2. The patient is given a rolled-up, partially-inflated, blood pressure cuff attached to a sphygmomanometer to squeeze.
3. A second cuff is applied to the arm, above the elbow, but it is not inflated.
4. Blood is taken for analysis of lactate and ammonium (Baseline).
5. The cuff on the arm is inflated to 120–140 mm of mercury, and the patient is instructed to squeeze the cuff rapidly (30–60 times per minute), trying as hard as possible to produce a pressure ≥ 100 mm of mercury. After 2 minutes, the cuff on the arm is deflated and the patient is instructed to relax.
6. Blood samples are obtained from the intravenous line for measurement of lactate and ammonium at 2, 5, 10, and 15 minutes after termination of the 2 minutes of ischemic exercise and deflation of the cuff on the arm.

treatment, that increased muscle protein breakdown to fuel gluconeogenesis is responsible.

Myoglobinuria (myophosphorylase deficiency phenotype)

The clinical course of *myophosphorylase deficiency* (McArdle disease or GSD V) is typical of a number of inherited defects of glycolysis presenting as exercise intolerance. It is characterized by the onset in early adulthood of severe muscle cramps shortly after the initiation of intense exercise; mild, sustained exercise, such as level walking, is well-tolerated. Typically, if the patient rests briefly, moderate levels of activity can be resumed without discomfort. This is the so-called 'second-wind' phenomenon. Presumably as the muscle converts to fatty acid oxidation in order to meet its energy needs, the requirement for glucose is decreased, and the cramps disappear. Episodes of cramping are often followed within hours by the development of wine-colored pigmentation of the urine (myoglobinuria) as a result of rhabdomyolysis. CPK levels are massively elevated and rise further during exercise. Rhabdomyolysis and resulting myoglobinuria occur in all myopathies arising as a result of defects in skeletal muscle energy metabolism. Rarely, it is severe enough to cause acute renal failure.

The normal accumulation of lactic acid in the course of an ischemic forearm exercise test does not occur, and the normal increase in plasma ammonium is exaggerated. The ischemic forearm exercise test (Table 2.8) involves the measurement of lactate and ammonium in blood collected from the antecubital vein before and after a defined period of vigorous exercise during which the circulation to the forearm is temporarily interrupted by application of a partially-inflated blood pressure cuff. In many patients, discomfort associated with the task forces interruption of the test before completion of the two minutes of vigorous exercise. In that case, blood samples for measurement of lactate and ammonium should continue to be collected as scheduled.

Muscle *phosphofructokinase* (PFK) *deficiency* (GSD VII) shares many features in common with myophosphorylase deficiency, including severe muscle cramping during short-term exercise, a 'second-wind' phenomenon, abnormal ischemic forearm exercise test, and myoglobinuria. However, onset in childhood is more common, the attacks of muscle cramps are generally more severe, and they are aggravated by ingestion of high-carbohydrate meals. Like patients with other inborn errors of glycolysis, patients with PFK deficiency generally show evidence of a compensated hemolytic anemia, and it may be associated with marked hyperuricemia. The disorder is more prevalent among Ashkenazi Jews and Japanese than in people of other ethnic groups.

Exercise intolerance of the 'myophosphorylase deficiency phenotype' occurs in patients with other glycolytic defects (Table 2.9), but these are rare. *Myoadenylate deaminase deficiency* is often clinically indistinguishable from myophosphorylase deficiency. However, the average age of onset is somewhat later, and the attacks of exercise-induced cramping tend to be less severe. CPK levels are increased in half the patients, and the electromyogram (EMG) is often normal. The ischemic forearm exercise test produces a normal increase in plasma lactate, but the normal increase in plasma ammonium does not occur. The diagnosis is confirmed by enzyme analysis or specific histochemical staining of muscle. In about half the patients with adenylate deaminase deficiency, the symptoms are due to secondary or acquired enzyme deficiency associated with other neuromuscular problems or with collagen vascular disease.

Myoglobinuria (CPT II phenotype)

In patients with myopathy resulting from defects in fatty acid oxidation, the muscle cramps and tenderness characteristically develop *after* periods of exercise, when the patient is actually at rest, and the muscle is drawing heavily on fatty acid oxidation to meet its energy requirements.

The main differences between the myophosphorylase deficiency and CPT II deficiency phenotypes are shown in Table 2.10. Most patients with *CPT II deficiency* present as young adults with a history of episodic muscle stiffness, pain, tenderness, weakness, and myoglobinuria precipitated by prolonged exercise, exposure to cold, fasting, or intercurrent infection. Patients do not experience a 'second-wind' phenomenon. Between attacks, they may be completely asymptomatic, though some experience residual muscle weakness and fatiguability. The

Table 2.9. *Inherited metabolic diseases presenting as muscle cramping or myoglobinuria.*

Disease	Clinical features	Diagnosis
Myophosphorylase deficiency phenotype		
Muscle phosphorylase deficiency (McArdle disease)	Muscle cramps during exercise, 'second-wind' phenomenon, normal pre-test lactate and no increase on ischemic forearm exercise test, elevated CPK, myogloginuria	Deficiency of phosphorylase in muscle
PFK deficiency	Muscle cramps during exercise, myoglobinuria, hyperuricemia (and gout), excessive increase of ammonium on ischemic forearm exercise test, compensated hemolytic anemia, elevated CPK, more common in Ashkenazi Jews and Japanese	Marked deficiency of PFK activity in muscle; half normal activities in erythrocytes
PGK deficiency	X-linked recessive, chronic hemolytic anemia, mental retardation, psychiatric problems	Deficiency of PGK in erythrocytes
PGAM deficiency	May be clinically indistinguishable from PFK deficiency	Deficiency of PGAM in muscle
LDH deficiency	May be clinically indistinguishable from PFK deficiency. No lactic acidosis, but marked hyperpyruvic acidemia during ischemic forearm exercise test	Deficiency of LDH-M subunit in erythrocytes
Myoadenylate deaminase deficiency	Post-exercise muscle cramps or myalgia, normal lactate response, but no increase in ammonium on ischemic forearm exercise test, elevated CPK in about 50%	Deficiency adenylate kinase on histochemical or biochemical analysis of skeletal muscle

CPT II deficiency phenotype

CPT II deficiency	Post-exercise cramps or myalgia, cold-induced muscle cramps and stiffness, increased CPK during fasting, normal lactate and ammonium responses but increased CPK on ischemic forearm exercise test, myoglobinuria	Deficiency of CPT II in fibroblasts
LCAD deficiency	Similar to CPT II deficiency, episodes of Reye-like encephalopathy, decreased plasma carnitine	Deficiency of LCAD in fibroblasts
SCHAD deficiency	Extremely rare, chronic muscle weakness with episodic acute deterioration and myoglobinuria, prominent myocardial involvement	Deficiency of SCHAD in muscle. Enzyme activity in fibroblasts is normal

Note: Abbreviations: CPT II, carnitine palmitoyltransferase II; LCAD, long-chain acyl-CoA dehydrogenase; SCHAD, short-chain 3-hydroxyacyl-CoA dehydrogenase; LDH, lactic dehydrogenase; PFK, phosphofructokinase; PGK, phosphoglycerate kinase; PGAM, phosphoglycerate mutase; CPK, creatine phosphokinase.

Table 2.10. *Differences between myophosphorylase deficiency and CPT II deficiency phenotypes.*

	Phenotype	
	Myophosphorylase	CPT II
Short-term intense exercise	Not tolerated	Well tolerated
Prolonged mild-moderate exercise	Well tolerated	Not tolerated
Second wind	Present	Absent
Effect of fasting	Beneficial	Detrimental
High carbohydrate-low fat diet	No benefit*	Beneficial

Note: *Although high carbohydrate dietary treatment is not beneficial in patients with myophosphorylase deficiency, a high-protein diet appears to be beneficial in some, and ingestion of glucose immediately before exercising often enhances exercise tolerance.
Abbreviation: CPT II, carnitine palmitoyltransferase II.
Source: Adapted from Di Mauro, Bresolin & Papadimitriou (1984).

CPK is elevated during attacks, but is generally normal at other times. Muscle biopsy shows lipid accumulation in many, though not all affected individuals. The myoglobinuria is severe enough in many patients to precipitate renal failure. The normal ketotic response to fasting (see Chapter 5) is blunted, though acute metabolic decompensation in older patients is rare. The diagnosis is confirmed by demonstrating deficiency of CPT II activity in fibroblasts.

Myopathy as a manifestation of multisystem disease (mitochondrial myopathies)

Progressive myopathy is often the principal manifestation of the multisystem involvement of diseases caused by defects in the mitochondrial ETC, though other systems are invariably involved. The extent and degree of involvement of various tissues and organs in patients with different mitochondrial ETC defects varies enormously, not only between unrelated patients, but even between patients within the same family. In some disorders, such as Leigh subacute necrotizing encephalopathy and Alpers disease (see section 'Chronic encephalopathy'), the myopathy is clinically mild compared with the effects of the disease on the CNS. However, in others, muscle weakness may be the presenting symptom and the multisystem nature of the condition is only appreciated after careful examination and laboratory studies. In most, the course of the disease is relentlessly progressive; in some, it is marked by episodes of acute deterioration superimposed on a background of chronic deterioration; and in a few, mostly

Table 2.11. *Some common features of conditions caused by mitochondrial mutations.*

Present in most mitochondrial conditions
Persistent lactic acidosis
Myopathy (weakness, hypotonia)
Failure to thrive; small stature
Psychomotor retardation
Seizures

Present in many mitochondrial conditions
Ophthalmoplegia or other oculomotor abnormalities
Retinal pigmentary degeneration
Hypertrophic cardiomyopathy
Cerebellar ataxia (progressive or intermittent)
Sensorineural deafness
Cardiac arrhythmias
Diabetes mellitus
Stroke (in children)
Renal tubular dysfunction
Respiratory abnormalities (periodic apnea and tachypnea)

young infants, spontaneous recovery occurs over a period of a few months. Most are associated with persistent lactic acidosis, though lactate levels are generally not > 10 mmol/L except during acute metabolic decompensation. The mode of inheritance may be autosomal recessive, autosomal dominant, X-linked, or mitochondrial (matrilineal). Among patients with disease due to mitochondrial mutations, a large proportion of them are *de novo* mutations, rather than inherited. However, the clinical symptomatology associated with mitochondrial mutations is often highly variable owing to the phenomenon of heteroplasmy (see Chapter 1), and other family members should be studied in detail before the mutation in a particular patient is concluded to be new. Characteristics which suggest that the myopathy is due to a mitochondrial ETC defect are shown in Table 2.11.

In spite of the enormous variability between patients with mitochondrial ETC defects, many patients with mitochondrial ETC defects exhibit groupings of clinical findings that have made it possible to identify some relatively distinct syndromes (Table 2.12).

Definitive investigation of this group of disorders requires muscle biopsy with histochemical studies, electron microscopy, and biochemical studies on mitochondrial electron transport in mitochondria isolated fresh from the tissue

Table 2.12. *Main clinical features of some relatively common mitochondrial syndromes.*

	KSS	MERRF	MELAS	NARP	LHON
Ophthalmoplegia	++++	0	0	0	0
Retinal degeneration	++++	0	0	++++	++++
Cerebellar dysfunction	+++	++++	0	+++	±
Psychomotor regression	++	++	+++	+	0
Myoclonus	0	++++	0	0	0
Seizures	+	+++	++++	++	0
Sensorineural deafness	+++	++	+	0	0
Cortical blindness ± hemiparesis (stroke)	0	0	++++	0	0
Renal tubular dysfunction	0	0	++	0	0
Skeletal abnormalities	0	0	0	0	±
Cardiac conduction defects	+++	0	0	0	+
Short stature	+++	++	+++	0	0
Diabetes mellitus	0	0	+	++	0
Lactic acidosis	++	++	+++	±	0
Common mutation	Large rearrangements	MTTK*MERRF8344	MTTL1*MELAS3243	MTATP6*NARP8993	MTND4*LHON11778
Positive family history	+	+++	++	+++	+++

Note: Abbreviations: KSS, Kearns-Sayre syndrome; MERRF, myoclonic epilepsy and ragged-red fibre disease; MELAS, Mitochondrial encephalomyopathy, lactic acidosis, and stroke-like episodes; NARP, neurodegeneration with ataxia and retinitis pigmentosa; LHON, Leber's hereditary optic neuropathy; +, present; ±, variably present; 0, not present. The abbreviation for each of the common mutations indicates the mitochondrial gene involved, the disease associated with the mutation, and the nucleotide number where the substitution has occurred.

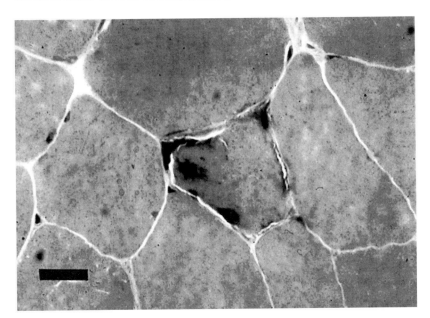

Fig. 2.7. Photomicrograph of skeletal muscle stained by the modified Gomori trichrome method showing ragged-red fibers. The bar represents 50 μm. (Courtesy of Dr. Venita Jay.)

(see Chapter 9). The presence of ragged-red fibers in skeletal muscle biopsies of the tissue stained by the modified Gomori trichrome stain (Figure 2.7) is a reflection of the proliferation and subsarcolemmal aggregation of mitochondria which is characteristic of many of the mitochondrial myopathies. Electron microscopic examination often confirms the presence of large aggregates of mitochondria. The mitochondria may be normal in appearance. However, they often show pathologic abnormalities in size, shape, and the number and orientation of cristae, and the presence of abnormal square or rectangular paracrystalline inclusions between the inner and outer mitochondrial membranes, or globular inclusions in the matrix. The tissue often contains excess glycogen and fat, sometimes giving the appearance of a 'lipid myopathy', such as is characteristic of the changes in patients with fatty acid oxidation defects.

The identification of specific mitochondrial mutations is a growing part of the investigation of mitochondrial disorders, including the mitochondrial myopathies. However, this is not yet routinely available except in a handful of centers doing basic research in the area.

Table 2.13. *Some inherited metabolic diseases characterized by psychiatric or severe behavioral abnormalities.*

Disease	Psychiatric/behavioral abnormality
Sanfilippo disease (MPS III)	Extreme hyperactivity, impulsivity, poor tolerance of frustration, aggressiveness, sleeplessness
Hunter disease (MPS II)	Extreme hyperactivity, impulsivity, poor tolerance of frustration, aggressiveness, sleeplessness
X-linked ALD	Social withdrawal, irritability, obsessional behavior, and rigidity
Late-onset MLD	Anxiety, depression, emotional lability, social withdrawal, disorganized thinking, poor memory, schizophrenia
Late-onset GM2 gangliosidosis	Acute psychosis with severe agitation, obsessional paranoia, hallucinations, stereotypic motor automatisms
Lesch-Nyhan syndrome	Severe self-mutilatory behavior
Porphyria	Chronic anxiety and depression, and marked restlessness, insomnia, depression, paranoia, and sometimes, hallucinations (during acute crises)
Wilson disease	Anxiety, depression, schizophrenia, manic-depressive psychosis, antisocial behavior
Cerebrotendinous xanthomatosis	Delusion, hallucinations, catatonia, dependency, irritability, agitation, and aggression
UCED	Periodic acute agitation, anxiety, hallucinations, paranoia
Homocystinuria due to MTHF reductase deficiency	Acute 'schizophrenia'
Adult-onset NCL	'Psychosis'

Note: Abbreviations: ALD, adrenoleukodystrophy; MLD, metachromatic leukodystrophy; UCED, urea cycle enzyme defects; MTHF, methylenetetrahydrofolate; NCL, neuronal ceroid lipofuscinosis.

Psychiatric problems

Some inherited metabolic disorders in which chronic progressive encephalopathy is prominent are characterized by severe behavior problems. For example, boys with Hunter disease (MPS II) and children with Sanfilippo disease (MPS III) exhibit particularly severe hyperactivity, impulsiveness, short attention span, poor tolerance of frustration, aggressiveness, and sleeplessness. In Sanfilippo disease, the extraordinarily disruptive behavior may be what brings the patient to medical attention. The implacable irritability of infants with

Krabbe globoid cell leukodystrophy is a prominent feature of the disease. Infants with hepatorenal tyrosinemia commonly exhibit acute episodes of extreme irritability, often accompanied by acute onset of reversible peripheral neuropathy, all attributable to the secondary porphyria which is a feature of the disease.

In many other inherited metabolic diseases, particularly late-onset disorders, the first indication of the onset of disease may be behavioral or personality changes (Table 2.13). The earliest signs of the disease in boys affected with X-linked adrenoleukodystrophy are often social withdrawal, irritability, obsessional behavior, and rigidity. Patients with adult-onset metachromatic leukodystrophy may present with subtle evidence of chronic organic brain syndrome, such as anxiety, depression, emotional lability, social withdrawal, disorganized thinking, and poor memory. In late-onset variants of GM2 gangliosidosis, the patient may present with a frank psychosis characterized by severe agitation, obsessional paranoia, hallucinations, and stereotypic motor automatisms. Personality changes are a common feature of Wilson disease, but usually only after the development of other neurologic manifestations of the disease. Three of our older pediatric patients with HHH syndrome have experienced periodic episodes of acute hallucinatory states lasting up to a few hours. The episodes generally occurred during periods of hyperammonemia, and the frequency of attacks decreased with improved metabolic control; however, their occurrence did not correlate well with the severity of the hyperammonemia.

Bibliography
Adams, R.D. & Lyon, G. (1982). *Neurology of Hereditary Metabolic Diseases of Children.* New York: McGraw-Hill Book Company.

Aicardi, J. (1993). The inherited leukodystrophies clinical overview. *Journal of Inherited Metabolic Diseases*, **16**, 733–43.

Batshaw, M.L. (1994). Inborn errors of urea synthesis. *Annals of Neurology*, **35**, 133–41.

Breningstall, G.N. (1986). Neurologic syndromes in hyperammonemic disorders. *Pediatric Neurology*, **2**, 253–62.

Breningstall, G.N. (1993). Approach to diagnosis of oxidative metabolism disorders. *Pediatric Neurology*, **9**, 81–90.

Chaves-Carballo, E. (1992). Detection of inherited neurometabolic disorders. A practical clinical approach. *Pediatric Clinics of North America*, **39**, 801–20.

CPC of the Massachusetts General Hospital (MGH 18-1979). (1979). A 34-year-old man with dysphasia. *New England Journal of Medicine*, **300**, 1037–45.

CPC of the Massachusetts General Hospital (MGH 2-1984). (1984). A 47-year-old man with right hemiplegia. *New England Journal of Medicine*, **310**, 106–14.

CPC of the Massachusetts General Hospital (MGH 7-1984). (1984). A 34-year-old man with progressive central nervous system dysfunction. *New England Journal of*

Medicine, **311**, 1170–7.

DiMauro, S., Bonilla, E., Zeviani, M., Nakagawa, M. & DeVivo, D.C. (1985). Mitochondrial myopathies. *Annals of Neurology*, **17**, 521–38.

DiMauro, S., Bresolin, N. & Papadimitriou, A. (1984). Fuels for exercise: Clues from disorders of glycogen and lipid metabolism. In *Neuromuscular Diseases*, ed. G. Serratrice *et al.*, pp. 45–50. New York: Raven Press.

Greene, C.L., Blitzer, M.G. & Shapira, E. (1988). Inborn errors of metabolism and Reye syndrome: differential diagnosis. *Journal of Pediatrics*, **113**, 156–9.

Hirano, M. & Pavlakis, S.G. (1994). Mitochondrial myopathy, encephalopathy, lactic acidosis, and strokelike episodes (MELAS): current concepts. *Journal of Child Neurology*, **9**, 4–13.

Hoffmann, G.F., Gibson, K.M., Trefz, F.K., Nyhan, W.L., Bremer, H.J. & Rating, D. (1994). Neurologic manifestations of organic acid disorders. *European Journal of Pediatrics*, **153**, S94–S100.

Munnich, A., Rötig, A., Chretien, D., Saudubray, J.M., Cormier, V. & Rustin, P. (1996). Clinical presentations and laboratory investigations in respiratory chain deficiency. *European Journal of Pediatrics*, **155**, 262–74.

Natowicz, M.R. & Bejjani, B. (1994). Genetic disorders that masquerade as multiple sclerosis. *American Journal of Medical Genetics*, **49**, 149–69.

Percy, A.K. (1992). Childhood metabolic disease with central nervous system involvement. *Current Opinion in Pediatrics*, **4**, 940–8.

Petty, R.K.H., Harding, A.E. & Morgan-Hughes, J.A. (1986). The clinical features of mitochondrial myopathy. *Brain*, **109**, 915–38.

3

Hyperphenylalaninemia and screening for PKU

Phenylketonuria (PKU)

PKU is the first described, and still the most common, autosomal recessive inborn error of metabolism causing disease in humans. Untreated, the condition is almost invariably associated with the development, within the first few months of birth, of characteristically severe mental retardation. But, if affected infants are treated from early infancy by carefully controlled dietary phenylalanine restriction, they grow up to be virtually indistinguishable from normal. Because a good outcome requires that treatment be started very early in infancy, large-scale screening programs were developed throughout the western world in the 1960s to identify affected infants in the newborn period. Experience with screening of newborns for PKU has led to the emergence of principles of genetic screening, which are reviewed in this chapter, and are now widely accepted as a model for the evaluation of genetic screening programs in general.

PKU is caused by hereditary deficiency of phenylalanine hydroxylase (PAH), which catalyzes the hydroxylation of phenylalanine to tyrosine (Figure 3.1). The enzyme activity occurs only in the liver, and the reaction requires tetrahydrobiopterin (BH4) as cofactor. Infants with so-called classical PKU, who have severe PAH mutations, have little residual hepatic phenylalanine hydroxylase activity and low dietary phenylalanine tolerance. On an unrestricted diet of prepared formula or breast milk, plasma phenylalanine levels are consistently above 1200 μmol/L.

Like all inherited metabolic diseases, the spectrum of biochemical and clinical severity of disease due to PAH mutations varies from one patient to another. Functionally subtle mutations, in which residual enzyme activity is presumably high, are associated with plasma phenylalanine levels (100–600 μmol/L) on unrestricted diets, and they are not associated with mental retardation. Infants in whom plasma phenylalanine levels are above 600 μmol/L, but below 1200 μmol/L, on an unrestricted diet, are considered to have intermediate variants of PKU. Many will suffer brain damage if they are not treated by dietary

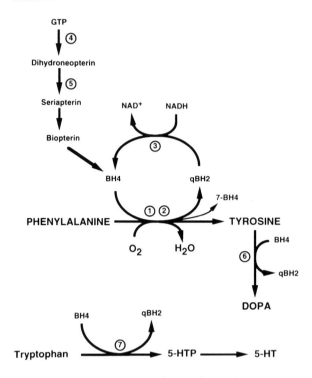

Fig. 3.1. The enzymic hydroxylation of phenylalanine to tyrosine, tyrosine to dihydroxyphenylalanine (DOPA), and tryptophan to 5-hydroxytryptophan (5-HTP).

The figure underscores the importance of tetrahydrobiopterin (BH4) in the biosynthesis of the neurotransmitter precursors, DOPA and 5-HTP. The enzymes shown are: **1**, phenylalanine hydroxylase; **2**, pterin-4α-carbinolamine dehydratase (PHS/PCD); **3**, dihydropteridine reductase (DHPR); **4**, GTP cyclohydrolase (GTPCH); **5**, 6-pyruvoyltetrahydropterin synthase (6-PTPS); **6**, tyrosine hydroxylase; **7**, tryptophan hydroxylase.

phenylalanine restriction. However, the risk of severe brain damage, and the degree of dietary phenylalanine restriction required to prevent it, are both lower than in infants with more complete defects.

PKU is a panethnic disease. However, the frequency of the different variants of the condition varies markedly between different ethnic groups: classical PKU is particularly common among northern Europeans, especially the Irish. It is rare among African blacks and Japanese, though it may be more common among Chinese. The benign variants are more common among Ashkenazi Jews and southern Europeans. It is transmitted as an autosomal recessive disorder.

The goal of dietary treatment of children with PKU is to prevent brain damage occurring from phenylalanine accumulation, while also supplying enough of the amino acid to support normal growth. This is achieved by maintaining plasma phenylalanine levels between 150 and 600 μmol/L, which requires frequent monitoring of plasma or blood phenylalanine levels with appropriate adjustments of the diet. The efficacy of dietary treatment is well established. However, in order to be effective, appropriate dietary management must be begun within one to three weeks of birth, before the development of symptoms of the disease and irreparable brain damage. The recognition that early detection and treatment of classical PKU resulted in the prevention of a particularly severe form of mental retardation, along with the discovery, in the early 1960s, of a simple, reliable, and inexpensive screening test based on the measurement of blood phenylalanine levels, led to the establishment of newborn screening programs throughout the western world. As a result, most infants with the disease are identified and treatment is instituted within a few weeks of birth. A 'positive PKU test' has become one of the ways in which an important inherited metabolic disease may present.

Screening for PKU

Screening for PKU was the first, formal, large-scale genetic screening initiative to be widely adopted in a direct attempt to ameliorate the impact of genetic disease, and the principles that have evolved since its introduction have served as a model for the development of numerous subsequent newborn screening programs, genetic and otherwise. The main principles, which were summarized by Charles Scriver in 1985 are:

- The specific reason for genetic screening should be clearly defined, whether the goal is medical intervention, as is the case with PKU, family planning, or research.
- Screening for medical intervention should be carried out in the context of an integrated program with the facilities, resources, and personnel to provide the necessary education and counselling for the population and participating health professions, the screening test, retrieval of individuals with positive screening tests, diagnostic confirmation, treatment, and evaluation of outcome.
- High-risk individuals should be detectable by a simple, inexpensive test which has high sensitivity (the proportion of affected infants with a positive screening test), specificity (the proportion of unaffected infants with a negative test), and predictive efficiency (ratio of true-positive to false-positive tests).

- The condition for which screening is contemplated should be medically significant in the population under consideration.
- When the goal of screening is treatment of disease, affected individuals should benefit significantly as a result of any medical intervention initiated on the basis of the screening procedure. To prove that treatment initiated early as a result of screening, rather than later when symptomatic, has a significant impact on the health and long-term well-being of the patient is sometimes difficult.
- Individuals should be informed of the goals, operation, and implications of the screening program, and they should have the right to refuse testing without prejudice.
- The outcome and impact of any screening program, regardless of the rationale for undertaking it in the first place, should be evaluated and the program modified, if necessary, based on the results of the evaluation.

Screening for the early detection of PKU is based on the demonstration of increased levels of phenylalanine in blood. The most commonly employed test is the Guthrie test, a bacterial inhibition assay of phenylalanine concentration in blood named after Robert Guthrie, the American physician-microbiologist who invented it. Only a few drops of blood, soaked into a special piece of filter paper and allowed to dry in air, are needed for the test. At the screening laboratory, small circles of blood-soaked filter paper are applied to the surface of agar plates containing a strain of *Bacillus subtilis* that requires phenylalanine for growth. The agar is impregnated with β-2-thienylalanine, a phenylalanine analogue which inhibits the utilization of phenylalanine by the organism. The amount of bacterial growth around the blood-soaked filter paper disks is proportional to the phenylalanine concentration in the blood. Quantitation of blood phenylalanine by the Guthrie test is unreliable when phenylalanine levels are below 200 or above 1500 μmol/L.

Like most biological assays, the Guthrie test requires careful standardization and the inclusion of suitable controls with each plate. Substances in the blood, such as antimicrobials, that interfere with bacterial growth will produce spuriously low phenylalanine concentrations. If the Guthrie test is done on or after the third day of life, the blood phenylalanine level in infants with classical PKU is high enough that the error caused by the presence of antimicrobials is trivial. However, if the test is done in the first few hours of life in an infant with classical PKU, or if the defect in phenylalanine metabolism is incomplete, the effect of the presence of antimicrobials might be sufficent to result in a spuriously negative screening test. In these circumstances, the test should be repeated within a few days.

An increasing number of screening laboratories are switching from the Guthrie test to chemical methods for the measurement of blood phenylalanine levels. The most common is a semi-automated spectrofluorometric method which yields more reliable results, particularly at very low and at very high phenylalanine concentrations. Chemical determination of phenylalanine levels is not affected by the presence of antimicrobial drugs or other substances which interfere with bacterial growth. Some laboratories rely on the semi-quantitative estimation of blood phenylalanine concentrations by thin-layer or paper chromatography. Enzymic methods for measurement of blood phenylalanine have also been developed, but they are not yet widely used. Many screening laboratories are considering switching to the more accurate chemical or enzymic screening tests owing to the growing trend to early discharge from hospital and the wide-spread use of the screening test to monitor the dietary treatment of children with PKU.

The sensitivity of PKU screening tests is high; few cases of PKU have been missed by failure of the test itself. The timing of the testing is important regardless of the test methodology. The blood phenylalanine concentration of infants with PKU at the time of birth is normal. Phenylalanine diffuses freely across the placenta, and metabolism of the amino acid by the mother prevents accumulation in the fetus. Within hours of birth, the plasma phenylalanine concentrations in infants with PKU rise, irrespective of feeding, to levels that are above normal. However, the levels encountered in older infants with untreated PKU do not develop for some days. Testing before the third day after birth increases the risk of missing infants with PKU, particularly infant girls. In countries where blood sampling for PKU screening is done in the hospitals of birth, the growing trend to early postnatal discharge has generated fears that infants with PKU will be missed by the screening process. Infants discharged from hospital before 24 hours of age should be tested immediately prior to discharge, regardless of age, and tested again within 10 days. Despite the potential for missing affected infants as a result of biologic or technical problems, most infants with PKU who have slipped through the screen seem to have done so as a result of administrative errors: failure to test, labeling errors, failure or inability to retrieve infants with positive tests.

The successful treatment of PKU requires carefully controlled dietary phenylalanine restriction for at least several years. This is possible only by careful dietary planning, the use of special low-phenylalanine dietary protein supplements, and frequent monitoring of blood phenylalanine levels. Most affected children are monitored by the use of the PKU screening test applied to blood samples taken at home, dried on appropriate filter-paper requisitions, and submitted to the treatment center for testing. Over the past two decades some important principles of management have emerged:

- Optimum outcome requires continuous maintenance of blood phenylalanine levels between 150 and 600 μmol/L.
- Treatment should be continued indefinitely. Although most of the brain damage occurring in children with untreated PKU appears to occur in the first few years of life, many show significant intellectual deterioration if dietary phenylalanine restriction is discontinued even after several years of therapy.
- Treatment of women with PKU during pregnancy is critical to the prevention of mental retardation in their offspring, whether or not the fetus has PKU, owing to the embryopathic effects of maternal hyperphenylalaninemia.
- The best results of treatment are obtained when it is centralized, generally in university-based treatment centers with close ties to the newborn screening program.

The outcome of screening for PKU and subsequent dietary treatment of the disease has been dramatic. Once appropriate dietary products and protocols were developed, by the late 1970s, the benefits of early, presymptomatic, detection, and carefully monitored dietary phenylalanine restriction, became obvious. Children with PKU, who would previously have almost certainly become severely mentally retarded by school age, were indistinguishable from normal. The observation that many exhibit subtle neuropsychologic deficits is currently being studied.

Biopterin defects

The enzymic conversion of phenylalanine to tyrosine by phenylalanine hydroxylase requires the participation of a cofactor, BH4 (Figure 3.1). BH4 is also required for the enzymic hydroxylation of tyrosine to dihydroxyphenylalanine (dopa) and of tryptophan to 5-hydroxytryptophan (5-HTP), precursors of the important neurotransmitters, dopamine and serotonin, respectively. Genetic defects in the synthesis or metabolism of BH4 cause hyperphenylalaninemia and are associated with severe mental retardation. Plasma phenylalanine levels in patients with biopterin defects are generally lower than the levels seen in children with classical PKU, and they also respond well to dietary phenylalanine restriction. Dietary treatment is often associated with an immediate improvement in the inattentiveness, irritability, and inactivity of symptomatic infants; however, the malignant neurodegenerative course of the disease is not significantly altered by dietary treatment alone. The severe clinical course in children with hereditary biopterin defects is presumably due to deficiencies of dopamine

Table 3.1. *Classification of inherited disorders of phenylalanine metabolism.*

Disorder	Characteristics
Classical phenylketonuria (PKU)	Plasma phenylalanine levels >1200 μmol/L on unrestricted diet
Atypical (mild) PKU	Plasma phenylalanine levels 600–1200 μmol/L on unrestricted diet
Persistent benign hyperphenylalaninemia	Plasma phenylalanine levels <600 μmol/L on unrestricted diet
Transient hyperphenylalaninemia	Early dietary phenylalanine intolerance becoming normal within a few weeks to months
Dihydropteridine reductase deficiency	Plasma phenylalanine levels 800–1200 μmol/L on unrestricted diet; requires treatment with diet and neurotransmitter precursors (dopa, Carbidopa, 5-HTP)
BH4 biosynthesis defects	Plasma phenylalanine levels 800–1200 μmol/L on unrestricted diet; requires treatment with BH4 and neurotransmitter precursors (dopa, Carbidopa, 5-HTP)
Maternal PKU	Low birth-weight, microcephaly, mental retardation, congenital heart disesae, and subtle facial dysmorphism in the offspring of women with PKU

Note: Abbreviations: BH4, tetrahydrobiopterin; 5-HTP, 5-hydroxytryptophan.

and serotonin in the brain. Plasma phenylalanine levels in infants with biosynthetic defects fall rapidly towards normal on treatment with exogenous BH4. However, BH4 does not cross the blood brain barrier. Infants with defects in BH4 biosynthesis or metabolism generally respond dramatically at first to treatment with L-dopa, Carbidopa, and 5-HTP; in some the response is sustained. In most, neurologic deterioration ultimately resumes in spite of therapy, resulting in severe neurologic impairment within a few years.

A classification of primary, inherited disorders of phenylalanine metabolism is shown in Table 3.1.

Secondary hyperphenylalaninemia

Most infants with positive PKU screening tests do not have PKU. The sensitivity and specificity of all tests currently used for population screening are close to

100%. However, the occurrence of a high proportion of false positive tests, a trade-off against high sensitivity, means that the predictive value of a positive test (the proportion of infants with a positive test who actually have PKU) may be as low as 10%. Usually, when the screening test is falsely positive, the blood phenylalanine level is only modestly to moderately elevated. Often, repeating the test produces normal results and the cause of the false positive result is not determined. However, in some common situations, the blood phenylalanine is persistently elevated, sometimes to levels seen in infants with mild PKU.

As many as half of the positive PKU screening tests are the result of transient hypertyrosinemia of premature newborns in which hepatic 4-hydroxyphenyl-pyruvate dioxygenase, the enzyme catalyzing the conversion of 4-hy-droxyphenylpyruvic acid to homogentisic acid, is immature. Increased plasma phenylalanine occurs as a secondary phenomenon in this situation. The condition is not due to an inborn error of metabolism, and it is not associated with any specific symptoms. Treatment of affected infants with large doses of ascorbic acid, coupled with reduction of dietary protein, usually results in rapid resolution of the condition.

Hepatocellular dysfunction, irrespective of the cause, is commonly associated with non-specific increases in plasma amino acid concentrations, particularly the concentrations of tyrosine and phenylalanine, producing a positive PKU screening test. The blood phenylalanine concentrations are never as high as those seen in infants with classical PKU, and the presence of elevated tyrosine levels, along with clinical and biochemical evidence of liver cell damage, suggests the origin of the problem. Rarely, infants with hepatorenal tyrosinemia, due to deficiency of fumarylacetoacetase activity (see Chapter 5), present with positive PKU screening tests.

Infants in neonatal intensive care units often have mild hyper-phenylalaninemia while receiving total parenteral nutrition (TPN). This is because of the increased phenylalanine content of TPN solutions. Tyrosine is so poorly soluble in aqueous solutions that delivery of nutritionally adequate amounts as the free amino acid is difficult. Manufacturers of TPN solutions overcome the difficulty meeting tyrosine requirements by increasing the phenylalanine content of the solutions. The effect is to deliver two to three times as much phenylalanine as an infant would receive from an unhydrolyzed milk-based formula. The resulting increase in blood phenylalanine levels is mild, transient, and harmless.

Investigative protocol
Protocols for the early identification of infants with biopterin defects are now considered a routine part of the investigation of hyperphenylalaninemia. A

suitable protocol for the investigation of a positive PKU screening test includes measures to:

- identify patients with hereditary phenylalanine hydroxylase deficiency;
- detect defects in tyrosine metabolism;
- detect defects in biopterin biosynthesis;
- detect dihydropteridine reductase (DHPR) deficiency.

This investigation can be done on an outpatient basis. Treatment by dietary phenylalanine restriction need not be delayed; however, the plasma phenylalanine level must still be elevated at least four to six times above normal at the time of the BH4 loading test (see below).

Initial quantitative analysis of plasma amino acids

This is done for accurate determination of the plasma phenylalanine concentration and determination of the concentration of tyrosine and other amino acids. In PKU, the tyrosine concentration is subnormal. In disorders of tyrosine metabolism associated with hyperphenylalaninemia, the tyrosine concentration is increased as well, and the phenylalanine to tyrosine ratio is low.

Blood DHPR assay

This is done to test for DHPR deficiency, which results in failure of regeneration of BH4 causing BH4 deficiency (Figure 3.1). DHPR is stable to drying and can be measured on dried blood spots like those used for screening for hyperphenylalaninemia.

Urinary biopterin/neopterin ratio and percentage BH4

Measurement of intermediates in BH4 biosynthesis serves to identify and localize defects in the process. Measurement must be done before the BH4 loading test (see below). Urine is collected into a collector with 100 mg of ascorbic acid powder and submitted without delay for biopterin analysis taking pains to ensure that it is stored frozen and protected from light.

BH4 loading test

This is another test for defects in BH4 biosynthesis. The plasma phenylalanine concentration must be elevated (>1000 μmol/L) in order to obtain interpretable results. Immediately after obtaining blood for quantitative analysis of plasma amino acids, administer BH4, 20 mg per kg body weight, by nasogastric tube, flushing the tube with water to ensure complete delivery of the medication. Obtain blood for quantitative analysis of plasma phenylalanine 6 and 12 hours after administering the BH4.

The sensitivity of BH4 loading tests is increased by combined oral loading with L-phenylalanine and BH4. The protocol has the advantages that it:

- can be performed on infants who have low plasma phenylalanine concentrations as a result of dietary phenylalanine restriction;
- eliminates the need to measure urinary pterins;
- is positive in infants with DHPR deficiency.

The test is performed by administration of L-phenylalanine (100 mg/kg), followed three hours later by administration of BH4 (20 mg/kg), and measurement of plasma phenylalanine levels before and 7 and 11 hours after the initial phenylalanine load. All infants with defects in the enzymic conversion of phenylalanine to tyrosine show marked increases in plasma phenylalanine levels after phenylalanine loading. In infants with defects in biopterin synthesis, the phenylalanine levels drop dramatically within four hours of BH4 loading. In infants with DHPR deficiency, plasma phenylalanine levels may also fall more rapidly than in infants with *PAH* mutations, but the drop is less abrupt than in defects of BH4 synthesis.

PAH *molecular genetic analysis*

The identification of specific *PAH* mutations is not currently regarded as part of the routine diagnosis of PKU, nor does it appear on its own to have much prognostic value. The molecular haplotype background on which the mutant *PAH* alleles occur appear to be more important than the mutations themselves. In northern Europeans, any combination of *PAH* mutations on haplotypes 2 or 3 is usually associated with severe PKU, whereas individuals with the same combinations of mutations on haplotypes 1 or 4 exhibit a wide range of disease severity. Because PAH is only expressed in the liver, mutation or molecular linkage analysis is the only way possible to prevent recurrence of the disease by prenatal diagnosis. Some of the principal mutations and haplotypes associated with PKU are shown in Table 3.2.

Although the majority of infants with PKU will come to attention as a result of screening programs, the trend to earlier discharge from hospital has increased the risk that affected newborns will be missed in the future, either as a result of the appropriate screening test not being done at all, or failure of the blood phenylalanine concentration to reach a level sufficiently elevated to trigger a positive test result. Various measures have been introduced in efforts to detect these infants, but they are, in general, less reliable than testing done as part of routine neonatal care. Owing to this growing trend for early postnatal discharge

Table 3.2. *Some common phenylalanine hydroxylase mutations and associated haplotypes in Caucasians.*

Mutation	Haplotype	Proportion of total* (%)
R408W	2	up to 65
IVS10nt546	6	up to 45
IVS12nt1	3	up to 35
R261Q	1	up to 35
M1V	2	up to 25
R408W	1	up to 20
Y414C	4	up to 20

Note: *Percentage of all mutant alleles bearing a specific mutation, depending on geographic location and ethnic group.

from hospital, infants with PKU will slip through the screening process unless compliance with re-testing several days later is complete. Infants with undetected PKU generally present at a few months of age with developmental delay, visual inattentiveness, inactivity, and delayed motor milestones. Affected infants also tend to be fair in complexion and often have an eczematoid rash. They emit a musty odor and are usually irritable in addition to being developmentally delayed. Infants with biopterin defects also show early microcephaly and seizures, features that generally develop only later in children with classical PKU.

Bibliography

Blau, N. (1988). Inborn errors of tetrahydrobiopterin metabolism. *Annual Review of Nutrition*, **8**, 185–209.

Dondt, J.-L. (1991). Strategy for the screening of tetrahydrobiopterin deficiency among hyperphenylalaninemic patients: 15 years experience. *Journal of Inherited Metabolic Diseases*, **14**, 117–27.

Guldberg, P., Levy, H.L., Koch, R., Berlin, Jr., C.M., Branxois, B., Henricksen, K.F. & Güttler, F. (1994). Mutation analysis in families with discordant phenotypes of phenylalanine hydroxylasae deficiency. Inheritance and expression of the hyper-phenylalaninemia. *Journal of Inherited Metabolic Disease*, **17**, 645–51.

Koch, R., Levy, H.L., Matalon, R., Rouse, B., Hanley, W.B., Trefz, F., et al. (1994). The international collaborative study of maternal phenylketonuria: status report 1994. *Acta Pediatrica*, Supplement 407, 111–19.

National Academy of Sciences (National Research Council). (1975). *Genetic Screening. Programs, Principles, and Research*. Washington: National Academy of Sciences.

Okano, Y., Eisensmith, R.C., Güttler, F., Lichter-Koneki, U., Koneki, D.S., Trefz, F.K.,

Dasovich, M., Wang, I., Henriksen, K., Lou, H. & Woo, S.C.L. (1991). Molecular basis of phenotypic heterogeneity in phenylketonuria. *New England Journal of Medicine*, **324**, 1232–8.

Scriver, C.R. (1985). Population screening: report of a workshop. In *Prevention of Physical and Mental Congenital Defects, Part B: Epidemiology, Early Detection and Therapy, and Environmental Factors*, ed. M. Marois, pp. 89–152. New York: Alan R. Liss, Inc.

Scriver, C. R., Eisensmith, R.C., Woo, S. L. C. & Kaufman, S. (1994). The hyperphenylalaninemias of man and mouse. *Annual Review of Genetics*, **28**, 141–65.

4

Metabolic acidosis

Metabolic acidosis is a common presenting or coincident feature of many inherited metabolic diseases. In some cases, the acidosis is persistent, though so mild that the generally recognized clinical signs, such as tachypnea, are absent or so subtle that they are missed. In other cases, the patient presents with an episode of acute, severe, even life-threatening, acidosis, and the underlying persistence of the condition is only recognized after resolution of the acute episode. Diagnostically, the most frustrating presentation is infrequent bouts of recurrent, acute acidosis separated by long intervals of apparent good health during which diagnostic tests show no significant abnormality. This is a particularly challenging situation.

Buffers, ventilation, and the kidney
The hydrogen ion concentration, $[H^+]$, of body fluids is maintained within very narrow limits by a combination of buffers, acting immediately, pulmonary ventilation to restore the capacity of blood buffers, and renal mechanisms to eliminate excess H^+.

Quantitatively, the most important buffers in blood are the proteins, both the plasma proteins and hemoglobin. Alterations in the concentrations of these proteins, particularly hemoglobin, may seriously compromise the capacity of the body to cope with sudden accumulation of acid. The buffering contributed by the equilibrium between HCO_3^- and H_2CO_3 is important because the capacity of the system is rapidly restored by elimination of H_2CO_3 through conversion to CO_2 and expulsion of the excess CO_2 by increased pulmonary ventilation.

The buffering properties of the bicarbonate–carbonic acid system are shown by the familiar Henderson-Hasselbach equation:

$$pH = pK' + \log \frac{[HCO_3^-]}{[H_2CO_3] + [CO_{2(d)}]}$$

$pK' =$ a constant = 6.10 in arterial blood; $CO_{2(d)}$ = concentration of dissolved CO_2.

In the presence of carbonic anhydrase, H_2CO_3 is rapidly converted to H_2O and CO_2. The concentration of H_2CO_3 is, therefore, directly proportional to the concentration of CO_2, which is a function of the partial pressure of CO_2, the $PaCO_2$, in blood. The pH and $PaCO_2$ of blood are easily measured, and with that information, the $[HCO_3^-]$ can be calculated. The equation is often re-written to show the relationship between its components in terms of the variables that are easily measured:

$$pH = pK' + \log \frac{[HCO_3^-]}{S \times PaCO_2}$$

$PaCO_2$ = partial pressure of CO_2 in arterial blood; S = a constant.

Without having to recall any specific numbers, one can easily see that an increase in $[H^+]$, in the absence of any other change, would cause a decrease in pH. However, association of the H^+ with HCO_3^- to form H_2CO_3 causes a decrease in $[HCO_3^-]$ and increase in $PaCO_2$, tending to restore the pH. Removal of the excess CO_2 by increased ventilation permits the association of more H^+ with HCO_3^- to form more H_2CO_3, though the total CO_2, and therefore the total buffer capacity of the system, is decreased in the process. Restoring the buffer capacity of the system requires removal of the excess H^+ by some other mechanism. This critical function is carried out by the kidney.

The kidney plays two important roles in acid-base balance: it conserves HCO_3^- (and sodium), and it secretes H^+. In the proximal convoluted tubule, 99% of filtered HCO_3^- is reabsorbed, along with sodium, amino acids and peptides, glucose, and phosphate. Loss of HCO_3^-, as a result of damage to the proximal convoluted tubule, decreases the buffering capacity of the bicarbonate-carbonic acid system. In the distal convoluted tubule of the nephron, H^+ is secreted by a mechanism involving exchange with K^+ and the production and secretion of NH_4^+ and glutamine. Decreased H^+–K^+ exchange, with increased K^+ losses in the urine, is the reason chronic metabolic alkalosis causes potassium depletion.

Metabolic acidosis is diagnosed by measurement of blood gases. The typical changes are:

- Decreased arterial blood pH, caused by accumulation of H^+.
- Decreased plasma bicarbonate, as excess H^+ is buffered by HCO_3^- with a shift in the equilibrium between HCO_3^- and H_2CO_3.
- Decreased $PaCO_2$, owing to compensatory hyperventilation.

If respiratory compensation is incomplete, resulting either from associated pulmonary disease or from respiratory failure, a mixed metabolic and respiratory acidosis develops, characterized by increased $PaCO_2$. Aggressive correction of metabolic acidosis, especially by administration of large amounts of sodium bicarbonate, is often accompanied by the development of a mixed respiratory and metabolic alkalosis as a result of persistence of central nervous system (CNS) acidosis after correction of the systemic acid-base disturbance.

Is the metabolic acidosis the result of abnormal losses of bicarbonate or accumulation of acid?

A glance at the Henderson-Hasselbach equation shows that the drop in pH occurring with metabolic acidosis may occur as a result of either abnormal losses of bicarbonate, or abnormal accumulation of H^+, generally in association with some organic anion. One way to tell the difference is to calculate the concentration of unmeasured anion, the anion gap, which is the difference between the plasma $[Na^+]$ and the sum of the plasma $[Cl^-]$ and $[HCO_3^-]$. The normal anion gap is 10–15 mEq/L. Albumin is quantitatively the most important unmeasured anion in plasma. Lactate, acetoacetate, 3-hydroxybutyrate, phosphate, sulfate, and other minor anions also contribute to the normal anion gap. When metabolic acidosis occurs as a result of bicarbonate losses, either because of renal tubular dysfunction or gastrointestinal losses from diarrhea, the anion gap is usually normal, in spite of decreased $[HCO_3^-]$, owing to an increase in the plasma $[Cl^-]$. Hyperchloremic acidosis is, therefore, one of the hallmarks of metabolic acidosis occurring as a result of abnormal bicarbonate losses.

Metabolic acidosis due to abnormal bicarbonate loss

A history of diarrhea is usually sufficient to distinguish hyperchloremic metabolic acidosis due to excessive gastrointestinal bicarbonate losses from that arising from renal tubular dysfunction. However, the situation may become confusing if the urine pH is discovered to be inappropriately high. The combination of acidosis and hypokalemia, owing to excessive gastrointestinal fluid and electrolyte losses, promotes renal ammonium production and excretion, increasing the urinary pH. By contrast, in patients with inappropriately high urinary pH as a result of renal tubular acidosis, the urine ammonium concentration is low. Urinary ammonium concentrations, which are difficult to measure directly, can be estimated by calculating the urine net charge (UNC): $[Na^+ + K^+] - [Cl^-]$ in urine. A negative UNC is taken as an indication of the presence of ammonium, suggesting the acidosis is the result of abnormal

Table 4.1. *Inherited metabolic diseases associated with renal tubular acidosis (RTA).*

Disease	Defect
Galactosemia	Galactose-1-phosphate uridyltransferase deficiency
Hereditary fructose intolerance	Fructose-1-phosphate aldolase deficiency
Hepatorenal tyrosinemia	Fumarylacetatoacetase deficiency
Cystinosis	Defect in cystine transport out of lysosomes
Glycogen storage disease, type I	Glucose-6-phosphatase deficiency
Congenital lactic acidosis	Cytochrome c oxidase deficiency
Wilson disease	Copper transporter defect
Vitamin D dependency	Cholecalciferol 1α-hydroxylase deficiency
Osteopetrosis with RTA	Carbonic anhydrase II deficiency
Lowe syndrome	Phosphatidylinositol-4,5-bisphosphate 5-phosphatase deficiency

gastrointestinal losses of bicarbonate (and potassium). This method for estimating urinary ammonium concentrations *does not apply* when the acidosis is the result of accumulation of organic anion.

The inappropriately high, though not necessarily alkaline, pH in patients with proximal renal tubular dysfunction is the result of excessive urinary losses of bicarbonate. In addition to bicarbonate, the reabsorption of amino acids, glucose, phosphate, and urate (*renal Fanconi syndrome*) is also impaired. The urine tests positive for glucose and reducing substances, and chromatographic analysis shows generalized amino aciduria (see Chapter 9). The plasma phosphate and urate concentrations are also below normal.

Renal Fanconi syndrome is a common manifestation of several inherited metabolic diseases (Table 4.1). However, the clinical signs of disease are generally dominated by other problems, rather than to the acidosis or renal disease *per se*. For example, the renal tubular problems in patients with galactosemia or hepatorenal tyrosinemia are usually discovered incidentally; they are rarely the presenting problem. In GSD I, and in hereditary fructose intolerance, the metabolic acidosis caused by massive accumulation of lactic acid is much more prominent than that caused by renal tubular dysfunction.

Chronic metabolic acidosis, whether it is attributable to bicarbonate losses or to accumulation of anion, is commonly associated with failure to thrive. Patients are often reported to be 'sickly' and to have exaggerated difficulties with apparently trivial intercurrent illnesses. Developmental delay is common, but rarely severe, and it is often noted to affect gross motor skills more than speech or socialization. When it is severe and persistent, as it is in infantile cystinosis, metabolic acidosis arising from proximal renal tubular disease is invariably associated with marked growth retardation. Excessive renal tubular loss of phosphate causes rickets.

Metabolic acidosis resulting from accumulation of organic anion

Metabolic acidosis resulting from accumulation of organic anion, caused by inborn errors of organic acid metabolism, is usually persistent. Clinically, it is commonly associated with marked failure to thrive. In addition, persistent, mild metabolic acidosis is often punctuated by intermittent episodes of acute metabolic decompensation. Acute metabolic acidosis causes tachypnea, often without obvious dyspnea. Breathing is rapid and deep, but often it is apparently effortless, and the severity of the respiratory distress may not be appreciated. Secondary hypoglycemia and hyperammonemia, along with accumulation of organic anion, commonly produce acute encephalopathy with anorexia and vomiting, lethargy, ataxia, and drowsiness progressing to stupor and coma (see Chapter 2). The accumulation of organic anion is often accompanied by a peculiar odor of the sweat or urine.

Diagnostically, the most important thing to do in patients presenting with metabolic acidosis and an increased anion gap is to identify the unmeasured anion. This is done by a combination of analysis of specific anions, such as lactate, 3-hydroxybutyrate and acetoacetate, and screening procedures, such as analysis of urinary organic acids (Figure 4.1) (see Chapter 9).

Lactic acidosis

Abnormal accumulation of lactic acid is by far the commonest cause of pathologic metabolic acidosis in children. In the majority of cases, it is caused by tissue hypoxia resulting from inadequate oxygen supply or poor circulation, so-called 'type A lactic acidosis'. It occurs in any situation in which the delivery of oxygen to tissues is impaired, such as shock, heart failure, congenital heart disease (especially that producing severe left outlet obstruction), or pulmonary hypertension. Lactic acidosis from hypoxemia may be very severe, with plasma lactate levels in excess of 30 mmol/L, and it is associated with an increase in the lactate to pyruvate ratio (L/P ratio) in plasma. The cause of the lactic acidosis is usually obvious, and the acidosis is generally reversed within minutes to a few hours by correction of the hypoxic state. The lactic acidosis associated with cardiomyopathy presents a special diagnostic challenge because the cardiomyopathy itself may be due to a primary inherited defect in lactate metabolism (see Chapter 6). A clinical classification of lactic acidosis is presented in Table 4.2.

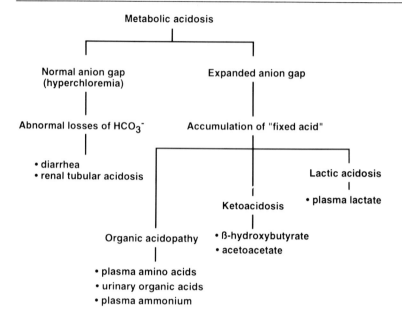

Fig. 4.1. Approach to the investigation of metabolic acidosis.

Lactate is a 'dead-end' metabolite: it is eliminated metabolically by the same route it is formed – through the formation of pyruvate. In addition to H⁺, the reaction involves two sets of substrates and products: pyruvate/lactate and NADH/NAD⁺. The conversion is catalyzed by lactate dehydrogenase (LDH), which is ubiquitous and catalyzes the forward and reverse reactions equally well, so that the equilibrium concentration of lactate is directly related to the concentration of pyruvate *and* the ratio of the concentrations of NADH and NAD⁺.

$$[\text{Lactate}] \propto [\text{Pyruvate}] \times [\text{H}^+] \times \frac{[\text{NADH}]}{[\text{NAD}^+]}$$

It follows that lactate accumulation may occur as a result of pyruvate accumulation or NADH accumulation, both tending to push the reaction to the right, or as a result of H⁺ accumulation.

Pyruvate accumulation

Pyruvate and lactate are the end products of *glycolysis*, the major source of energy when availability of oxygen is low and in tissues, like erythrocytes, that do not

Table 4.2. *Clinical classification of lactic acidosis.*

Acquired	Inborn errors of metabolism
Hypoxemia	*Primary*
Circulatory collapse	Defects of pyruvate metabolism
Shock	PDH deficiency
Congestive heart failure	Pyruvate carboxylase deficiency
Severe systemic disease	Defects of NADH oxidation
Liver failure	Mitochondrial ETC defects
Kidney failure	*Secondary*
Diabetic ketoacidosis	Disorders of gluconeogenesis
Acute pancreatitis	GSD, type I
Acute leukemia	HFI
Intoxication	PEPCK deficiency
Ethanol	Fructose-1,6-diphosphatase deficiency
Methanol	Fatty acid oxidation defects
Ethylene glycol	Defects of biotin metabolism
Oral hypoglycemic drugs	Biotinidase deficiency
Acetylsalicylic acid	Holocarboxylase synthetase deficiency
Nutritional deficiency	Defects of organic acid metabolism
Thiamine deficiency	HMG-CoA lyase deficiency
	Propionic acidemia
	Methylmalonic acidemia
	Others

Note: Abbreviations: PDH, pyruvate dehydrogenase; GSD, glycogen storage disease; HFI, hereditary fructose intolerance; PEPCK, phosphoenolpyruvate carboxykinase; HMG-CoA, 3-hydroxy-3-methylglutaryl-CoA.
Source: Modified from Lehotay & Clarke (1995).

contain mitochondria. Many of the reactions are freely reversible and contribute equally well to *gluconeogenesis*, the process by which glucose is produced from pyruvate and amino acids (see Chapter 5). Although the sequence of reactions and the regulation of the rate and direction of metabolic flux is complicated, clinically important aspects of the process can be summarized in a few generalizations and the whole treated as a 'black box'. The key features of glycolysis are:

- It is a cytoplasmic process.
- Each molecule of glucose (six carbons), which is uncharged, is converted to two molecules of pyruvic acid (three carbons each), which are negatively charged.

Table 4.3. *Effect of various metabolic intermediates on glycolytic flux.*

Increase glycolytic flux	Decrease glycolytic flux
cAMP	ATP
AMP	Citrate
ADP	Fatty acids
Inorganic phosphate	NADH
Fructose-2,6-bisphosphate	Acetyl-CoA
Glucose-6-phosphate	

- It results in the net production of two molecules of ATP per molecule of glucose.
- Overall flux is increased by an intracellular energy deficit and is decreased by signals indicating the concentrations of high energy compounds, like ATP, are adequate (Table 4.3).
- It produces various intermediates, such as glycerol, required for the synthesis of compounds like triglyceride.

Among the inherited metabolic diseases, lactic acidosis due to pyuvate accumulation may occur as a result of *increased pyruvate production* by increased glycolytic flux. Increased pyruvate production is the mechanism of the lactic acidosis in patients with GSD I, or hereditary fructose intolerance, as a consequence of increased intracellular concentrations of stimulatory phosphorylated intermediates, like fructose-2,6-bisphosphate and fructose-1,6-bisphosphate, respectively.

Lactic acidosis also occurs as a consequence of *decreased oxidation of pyruvate.* Pyruvate, produced from glycolysis, or from the transamination of alanine, is either oxidized to acetyl-CoA, in a reaction catalyzed by the pyruvate dehydrogenase complex (PDH), or it is carboxylated, in a reaction catalyzed by the biotin-containing enzyme, pyruvate carboxylase (PC), to form oxaloacetate, fueling the tricarboxylic acid (TCA) cycle (Figure 4.2). Whether PDH or PC activity predominates at any particular moment is, as one might expect, determined by the energy needs of the cell. In general, PDH is stimulated by signals indicating an increased need for energy, such as low ATP/ADP ratios; PC is stimulated by indications, such as increased acetyl-CoA levels, that the concentration of TCA intermediates, particularly oxaloacetate, is too low to support continued operation of the cycle.

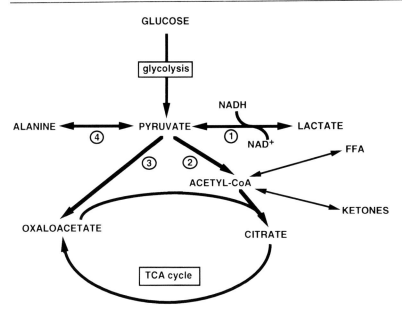

Fig. 4.2. Metabolic sources and fates of pyruvate.
The enzymes involved in pyruvate metabolism are: **1**, lactate dehydrogenase; **2**, pyruvate dehydrogenase complex; **3**, pyruvate carboxylase; **4**, alanine aminotransferase.

PDH deficiency

Persistent lactic acidosis is a prominent feature of PDH deficiency. PDH is a huge multicomponent enzyme complex made up of multiple units of four enzymes: pyruvate decarboxylase (E_1, 30 units), dihydrolipoyl transacetylase (E_2, 60 units), dihydrolipoyl dehydrogenase (E_3, 6 units), and protein X (6 units). Enzyme activity is regulated in part by phosphorylation (inactivation)–dephosphorylation (activation), reactions catalyzed by PDH kinase and PDH phosphatase, respectively. Most patients with PDH deficiency have mutations of the X-linked $E_1\alpha$ subunit of the pyruvate decarboxylase component of the enzyme complex. Nonetheless, males and females are equally represented, except among those patients with the relatively benign form of the disease which is characterized by intermittent ataxia (see Chapter 2).

The clinical course of PDH deficiency is highly variable. The disease may present in the newborn period as severe persistent lactic acidosis (see Chapter 8) terminating in death within a few weeks or months. This variant of the disease is often associated with agenesis of the corpus callosum. Most children with PDH deficiency present later in infancy with a history of psychomotor retardation, hypotonia, failure to thrive, and seizures. The course of the disease is often punctuated by bouts of very severe lactic acidosis, often precipitated by intercurrent infections. Some show subtly dysmorphic facial features. Other patients present with classical Leigh disease (see Chapter 2).

Plasma lactate levels in PDH deficiency are persistently elevated, and the acidosis is generally made worse by ingestion of carbohydrate. However, the L/P ratio is characteristically normal. The plasma alanine level is elevated, a reflection of increased pyruvate concentrations. Urinary organic acid analysis in patients with $E_1\alpha$ defects is unremarkable apart from the presence of excess lactate and some 2-hydroxybutyrate, an organic acid found in the urine of patients with severe lactic acidosis, regardless of the cause. The diagnosis is confirmed by demonstrating PDH deficiency in fibroblasts. Rarely, the PDH deficiency may be the result of a defect in the E_3 component (lipoamide dehydrogenase) of the enzyme complex. Clinically, affected patients are indistiguishable from patients with $E_1\alpha$ defects, though presentation in the newborn period has never been reported. Because both branched-chain 2-ketoacid dehydrogenase and 2-ketoglutarate dehydrogenase also contain the same E_3 subunit as PDH, patients with E_3 defects have elevated plasma levels of branched-chain amino acids, though not as high as in maple syrup urine disease (MSUD), and the urinary organic acid analysis shows increased concentrations of 2-ketoglutarate, 2-hydroxyglutarate, and 2-hydroxyisovalerate. A small number of patients with classical Leigh disease have been found to have PDH phosphatase deficiency.

Although a few vitamin-responsive variants of PDH deficiency have been reported, treatment of this group of disorders is usually unsatisfactory. However, boys with the benign variant often do better on a high fat, low carbohydrate diet. The lactic acidosis in some patients is relieved to some extent by treatment with the pyruvate analogue, dichloroacetate, which increases PDH activity by inhibiting PDH kinase.

PC deficiency

Persistent lactic acidosis is also a prominent feature of PC deficiency. PC is a biotin-dependent enzyme which catalyzes the carboxylation of pyruvate to form oxaloacetate. It is dependent for activity on the presence of acetyl-CoA. In addition to its role in fueling the TCA cycle, PC catalyzes the first, and most important, reaction in gluconeogenesis (see Chapter 5).

PC deficiency is very rare. The most common variant of the disorder (type A) commonly presents in the first few months of life with a history of psychomotor

Table 4.4. *Urinary organic acids in multiple carboxylase deficiency.*

Enzyme deficiency		
3-Methylcrotonyl-CoA dehydrogenase	**Propionyl-CoA carboxylase**	**Pyruvate carboxylase**
3-Methylcrotonate	Propionate	**Lactate**
3-Methylcrotonylglycine	**3-Hydroxypropionate**	3-Hydroxybutyrate
3-Hydroxyisovalerate	**Methylcitrate**	Acetoacetate
	Tiglylglycine	

Note: Bold indicates those compounds which are consistently present or present in high concentrations in the disease.

retardation and signs of intermittent acute metabolic acidosis. Despite the central role PC plays in gluconeogenesis, hypoglycemia is not as a rule a prominent feature of the disease. The majority of patients in North America have been Amerindian. The L/P ratio is normal. The plasma alanine and proline levels are elevated. Urinary organic acid analysis shows elevated concentrations of lactate and 2-ketoglutarate.

Patients with the severe form of PC deficiency (type B) present in the newborn period with chronically severe lactic acidosis culminating in death within a few months. In contrast to type A patients, the L/P ratio is elevated. In addition to the biochemical abnormalities found in type A disease, affected infants are moderately hyperammonemic, and the concentrations of citrulline, lysine, and proline are increased in plasma. The diagnosis is confirmed by measuring PC activity in peripheral blood leukocytes or in fibroblasts.

Multiple carboxylase deficiency

Patients with multiple carboxylase deficiency, either because of holocarboxylase synthetase deficiency or biotinidase deficiency, is associated with lactic acidosis which is the result of deficiency of PC, one of the four biotin-dependent enzymes affected in the disease. *Holocarboxylase synthetase deficiency* is rare and usually presents within the first few weeks of birth with signs of acute metabolic acidosis accompanied by hyperammonemia. Feeding problems, failure to thrive, hypotonia, psychomotor retardation, peculiar odor, and seizures are also common and prominent features of the disease. *Biotinidase deficiency* is more common than holocarboxylase synthetase deficiency, and clinical presentation is generally later in infancy. Presentation is usually with psychomotor delay, hypotonia, myoclonic seizures, and acute metabolic acidosis. Most patients also have a seborrheic skin rash and at least partial alopecia; many have conjunctivitis, fungal infections, and other evidence of impaired resistance to infection. Some show evidence of optic atrophy, sensorineural hearing loss, and ataxia.

The urinary organic acid profile in these disorders reflects the deficiencies of the three biotin-dependent mitochondrial carboxylases involved (Table 4.4). The organic aciduria in these disorders is variable, particularly biotinidase deficiency, in which the organic acids in urine may be normal. The diagnosis of biotinidase deficiency can be confirmed by enzyme assay on dried blood spots using synthetic chromogenic or fluorogenic substrates; the determination of holocarboxylase synthetase is based on the effect of biotin treatment on the activity of the mitochondrial carboxylases in peripheral blood leukocytes or cultured fibroblasts. Both forms of multiple carboxylase deficiency respond to treatment with large doses of oral biotin, though the response and ultimate outcome tends to be better for infants with holocarboxylase synthetase deficiency.

NADH accumulation

NADH production, like pyruvate production, is increased by any process that increases glycolytic flux. Ignoring for the moment problems of intracellular compartmentation and the complex matter of NADH transport within the cell, the principal route of NADH disposal by oxidation is by intramitochondrial electron transport linked to ATP generation – the main energy-producing process in the body. In this process, the final electron acceptor is oxygen, and any condition causing local or systemic hypoxia will cause NADH accumulation and lactic acidosis. NADH accumulation, whether the result of increased production or decreased oxidation, causes lactic acidosis by pushing the pyruvate–lactate equilibrium toward lactate. Therefore, defects of NADH oxidation, including inborn errors of the mitochonrial electron transport chain (ETC), are typically characterized by increased L/P ratios. The laboratory investigation of mitochondrial ETC defects is discussed in Chapter 9.

A rapidly growing number of patients with disease caused by ETC defects is being reported. Although many are associated with lactic acidosis as a result of NADH accumulation, the acidosis is generally not severe and is rarely the problem that brings the patient to medical attention. Instead, most present with one or more of: psychomotor retardation, skeletal myopathy, cardiomyopathy, hepatocellular dysfunction, or retinal degeneration, although other conditions have been associated with mitochondrial mutations, including *diabetes mellitus* (see Chapter 2). There is considerable overlap in the relationship between the type of mutation or the ETC complex affected and the clinical pattern of disease

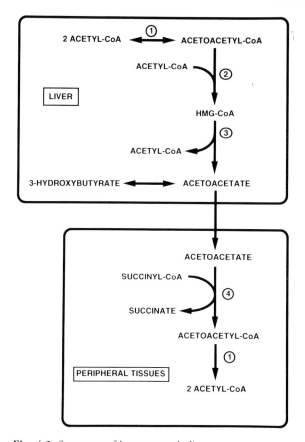

Fig. 4.3. Summary of ketone metabolism.
The reactions involved in ketone production and oxidation are: **1**, acetoacetyl-CoA thiolase; **2**, 3-hydroxy-3-methylglutaryl-CoA (HMG-CoA) synthetase; **3**, HMG-CoA lyase; **4**, succinyl-CoA:3-ketoacid CoA transferase (SCOT).

among patients with mitochondrial ETC defects. For example, Leigh disease has been found associated with defects in Complex I, Complex IV, Complex V, as well as PC deficiency and PDH deficiency. In this situation, the clinical presentation provides very little insight into the nature of the underlying genetic defect.

Ketoacidosis
Increased fatty acid oxidation results in the production of large amounts of acetyl-CoA (see Chapter 5). Excess acetyl-CoA condenses in the liver to produce

ketones (3-hydroxybutyrate and acetoacetate) which are exported via the circulation to be taken up and oxidized by peripheral tissues, including the brain (Figure 4.3). This is one of the most important adaptations to starvation because the ability of tissues, such as the brain, which normally derive much of their energy from glucose oxidation, to utilize ketones for energy, spares the glucose for use by tissues, such as erythrocytes, which cannot derive energy from non-glucose energy substrates. Defects in ketone utilization cause ketoacidosis.

Ketoacidosis, sometimes severe, is a prominent secondary phenomenon in several inherited metabolic diseases, such as MSUD, organic acidopathies (e.g., methylmalonic acidemia, propionic acidemia, isovaleric acidemia, holocar-boxylase synthetase deficiency), glycogen storage diseases (e.g., GSD type III, hepatic phosphorylase deficiency, phosphorylase kinase deficiency, glycogen synthase deficiency), and disorders of gluconeogenesis (e.g., pyruvate carboxylase deficiency, fructose-1,6-diphosphatase deficiency, phosphoenolpyruvate car-boxykinase deficiency). Primary disorders of ketone utilization are rare.

Mitochondrial acetoacetyl-CoA thiolase deficiency (β-ketothiolase deficiency)

β-Ketothiolase deficiency is characterized by the onset between one and two years of age of episodic attacks of severe ketoacidosis and encephalopathy, generally precipitated by intercurrent illness or fasting, sometimes associated with hyperammonemia. The response to treatment with intravenous glucose is characteristically brisk, and between episodes of metabolic decompensation, patients are typically completely well. Urinary organic acid analysis at the time of metabolic decompensation shows the presence of 2-methyl-3-hydroxybutyrate, 2-methylacetoacetate, 2-butanone, and tiglylglycine – all derived from the intermediary metabolism of isoleucine (Figure 4.4), as well as huge amounts of 3-hydroxybutyrate and acetoacetate. Definitive diagnosis requires demonstra-tion of specific deficiency of potassium-stimulated enzyme activity, preferably using 2-methylacetoacetyl-CoA as substrate. Cytosolic acetoacetyl-CoA thiolase deficiency is very rare. It is characterized by severe psychomotor retardation and hypotonia, a reflection perhaps of the importance of the enzyme in sterol and isoprenoid biosynthesis.

Succinyl-CoA:3-ketoacid CoA-transferase (SCOT) deficiency

Only a few patients with SCOT deficiency have ever been studied. All presented early in life with life-threatening bouts of severe ketoacidosis. Unlike patients with β-ketothiolase deficiency, who may be to all appearances completely normal between episodes of ketoacidosis, patients with SCOT deficiency are persistently

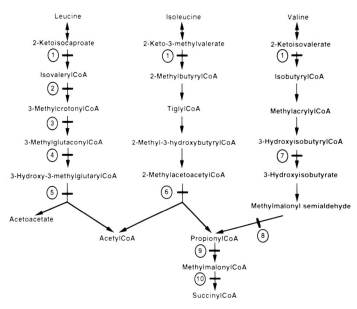

Fig. 4.4. Branched-chain amino acid metabolism.
The various enzymes shown are: **1**, branched-chain 2-ketoacid decarboxylase; **2**, isovaleryl-CoA dehydrogenase; **3**, 3-methylcrotonyl-CoA carboxylase; **4**, 3-hydroxy-3-methylglutaryl-CoA (HMG-CoA) synthetase; **5**, HMG-CoA lyase; **6**, 2-methylacetoacetate thiolase; **7**, 3-hydroxyisobutyryl-CoA deacylase; **8**, methylmalonyl semialdehyde dehydrogenase; **9**, propionyl-CoA carboxylase; **10**, methylmalonyl-CoA mutase.

ketotic between episodes of metabolic decompensation. The urinary organic acid analysis shows large amounts of 3-hydroxybutyrate and acetoacetate.

Organic aciduria

The development of rapid, accurate, and technically relatively easy and inexpensive techniques for the analysis of low molecular weight organic acids in physiologic fluids, like urine, has led to the discovery of a large number of new inherited metabolic diseases. A number of these present as acute, chronic, or acute-on-chronic metabolic acidosis, and urinary organic acid analysis is a logical and important aspect of the diagnostic investigation. However, for some organic acidopathies, clinical signs of metabolic acidosis may be so subtle that they are completely obscured by symptoms referable to the nervous system, heart, liver, kidneys, or other systems. To limit the application of organic acid analysis to

Table 4.5. *Organic acidurias.*

Urinary organic acids	Enzyme deficiency	Distinguishing clinical features
2-Ketoisocaproate, 2-hydroxycaproate, 2-keto-3-methylvalerate, 2-ketoisovalerate, 2-hydroxyisovalerate	Branched-chain 2-ketoacid decarboxylase	MSUD: Acute encephalopathy, ketosis, psychomotor retardation
Lactate, 2-ketoglutarate, 2-ketoisocaproate, 2-hydroxycaproate, 2-keto-3-methylvalerate, 2-ketoisovalerate, 2-hydroxyisovalerate	Lipoamide dehydrogenase	Psychomotor retardation, chronic lactic acidosis with acute exacerbations
3-Methylglutaconate, 3-hydroxyisovalerate, 3-methylglutarate, 3-hydroxybutyrate, acetoacetate	3-Methylglutaconyl-CoA hydratase	3-Methylglutaconic aciduria, type I: mild psychomotor retardation, hypoglycemia, ketoacidosis
3-Methylglutaconate, 3-methylglutarate, 2-ethylhydracrylate	Unknown	Barth syndrome (3-methylglutaconic aciduria, type II): X-linked, cardiomyopathy, skeletal myopathy, chronic neutropenia
3-Methylglutaconate, 3-methylglutarate	Unknown	Costeff optic atrophy syndrome (3-methylglutaconic aciduria, type III): optic atrophy, severe psychomotor retardation, choreoathetosis, spasticity, seizures
3-Methylglutaconate, 3-methylglutarate, lactate, TCA cycle intermediates	Mitochondrial ATP-synthase	3-Methylglutaconic aciduria, type IV: severe multi-organ disease, congenital malformations, clinically heterogenous, including Pearson mitochondrial deletion syndrome

Metabolites	Enzyme	Clinical features
3-Hydroxy-3-methylglutarate, 3-methylglutaconate, 3-methylglutarate, 3-hydroxyisovalerate	HMG-CoA lyase	Episodic severe metabolic acidosis with encephalopathy, hypoglycemia ± hyperammonemia
Mevalonate	Mevalonate kinase	Psychomotor retardation, dysmorphism, cataracts, hepatosplenomegaly, lymphadenopathy, anemia, chronic diarrhea, arthralgia, fever, skin rash
Isovalerylglycine, 3-hydroxyisovalerate, lactate, 3-hydroxybutyrate, acetoacetate	Isovaleryl-CoA dehydrogenase	Severe metabolic acidosis, hyperammonemia, neutropenia, thrombocytopenia, odor of sweaty feet
2-Methyl-3-hydroxybutyrate, 2-methylacetoacetate, 2-butanone, 3-hydroxybutyrate, acetoacetate, tiglylglycine	Mitochondrial acetoacetyl-CoA thiolase	Episodic severe ketoacidosis.
3-Methylcrotonate, 3-methylcrotonylglycine, 3-hydroxyisovalerate	3-Methylcrotonyl-CoA carboxylase	Episodic severe ketoacidosis, hypoglycemia
3-Methylcrotonate, 3-methylcrotonylglycine, 3-hydroxyisovalerate, propionate, 3-hydroxypropionate, methylcitrate, tiglylglycine, lactate, 3-hydroxybutyrate and acetoacetate	(a) Holocarboxylase synthetase or (b) Biotinidase	(a) Metabolic acidosis, hyperammonemia, thrombocytopenia, peculiar odor, seizures, ataxia, (skin rash, alopecia) (b) Psychomotor delay, hypotonia, myoclonic seizures, metabolic acidosis, seborrheic skin rash, alopecia
Ethylmalonate, methylsuccinate, butyrylglycine, isovalerylglycine, 2-methylbutyrylglycine	2-Methylbranched-chain acyl-CoA dehydrogenase deficiency	Spastic diplegia, orthostatic acrocyanosis, chronic diarrhea, psychomotor retardation, lactic acidosis

Table 4.5. (*Cont.*)

Urinary organic acids	Enzyme deficiency	Distinguishing clinical features
Ethylmalonate, 2-methylbutyrylglycine, isobutyrylglycine, isovalerylglycine	Cytochrome *c* oxidase	Psychomotor retardation, encephalopathy, ataxia, spasticity
L-2-Hydroxyglutarate	Unknown	Ataxia, dysarthria, psychomotor retardation, ± seizures
D-2-Hydroxyglutarate	D-2-Hydroxyglutarate dehydrogenase	Psychomotor retardation, seizures
Methylmalonate, methylcitrate, 3-hydroxybutyrate, acetoacetate	Methylmalonyl-CoA mutase or Cobalamin defects	Severe metabolic acidosis, hyperammonemia, neutropenia, thrombocytopenia
3-Hydroxyisobutyrate, lactate	3-Hydroxyisobutyryl-CoA dehydrogenase	Episodic ketoacidosis, facial dysmorphism, cerebral dysgenesis, hypotones, failure to thrive, episodes of acidosis
4-Hydroxybutyrate, 3,4-dihydroxybutyrate	Succinic semialdehyde dehydrogenase	Psychomotor retardation, hypotonia, ataxia, choreoathetosis
Fumarate	Unknown	Psychomotor retardation
Propionate, 3-hydroxypropionate, propionylglycine, methylcitrate, tiglylglycine, 3-hydroxybutyrate, acetoacetate	Propionyl-CoA carboxylase	Severe metabolic acidosis, hyperammonemia, neutropenia, thrombocytopenia
Malonate	Malonyl-CoA decarboxylase	Psychomotor retardation ± cardiomyopathy
L-Glycerate, oxalate	D-Glycerate dehydrogenase	Urolithiasis, urinary tract infections, renal colic

Enzyme/Deficiency	Clinical features	Metabolites
Peroxisomal alanine:glyoxylate aminotransferase (type I)	Urolithiasis, nephrocalcinosis, peripheral neuropathy, anemia, arthropathy, progressive renal failure	Oxalate, glycolate
Medium-chain acyl-CoA dehydrogenase	Recurrent Reye-like encephalopathy, sudden unexpected death	Medium-chain dicarboxylic acids (adipate, suberate, sebacate), 5-hydroxyhexanoate, 7-hydroxyoctanoate, hexanoylglycine, phenylpropionylglycine, octanoylcarnitine
Short-chain acyl-CoA dehydrogenase	Skeletal myopathy, cardiomyopathy, failure to thrive, metabolic acidosis, neutropenia	Ethylmalonate, methylsuccinate, adipate, butyrylglycine
Long-chain acyl-CoA dehydrogenase	Cardiomyopathy, skeletal myopathy, exercise intolerance with myoglobinuria, Reye-like episodes of acute encephalopathy	Medium-chain dicarboxylic acids, dodecandioate, tetradecandioate
Long-chain 3-hydroxyacyl-CoA dehydrogenase	Cardiomyopathy, variable skeletal myopathy, intermittent acute hepatocellular dysfunction	Medium-chain dicarboxylic acids, 3-hydroxydodecandioate, 3-hydroxydodecendioate, 3-hydroxytetradecandioate, 3-hydroxytetradecendioate
Glutaryl-CoA dehydrogenase	Progressive dystonia, choreoathetosis, gross motor retardation, intermittent ketoacidosis and acute encephalopathy	Glutarate, 3-hydroxyglutarate
Electron transport flavoprotein (ETF) or ETF dehydrogenase (multiple acyl-CoA dehydrogenase deficiency)	Facial dysmorphism, cerebral dysgenesis, cystic kidneys (severe), or intermittent severe ketoacidosis, hyperammonemia, acute encephalopathy, failure to thrive (mild)	Glutarate, 2-hydroxyglutarate, ethylmalonate, adipate, suberate, sebacate, dodecanedioate, isovalerylglycine, hexanoylglycine

Table 4.5. (*Cont.*)

Urinary organic acids	Enzyme deficiency	Distinguishing clinical features
5-Oxoproline (pyroglutamate)	Glutathione synthetase	Hemolytic hypochromic, microcytic anemia
4-Hydroxycyclohexylacetate	4-Hydroxyphenylpyruvate oxidase	Hawkinsinuria: autosomal dominant, intermittent metabolic acidosis in infancy
N-Acetylaspartate	Aspartoacylase	Canavan syndrome: severe, progressive psychomotor retardation, macrocephaly, seizures
Orotate	(a) UMP synthase or (b) Various defects in urea biosynthesis	(a) Megaloblastic anemia, urolithiasis, failure to thrive, psychomotor retardation (b) See Chapter 2
Uracil, thymine	Dihydropyrimidine dehydrogenase	Uncertain. Increased susceptibility to 5-fluorouracil toxicity

Note: Abbreviations: MSUD, maple syrup urine disease; TCA, tricarboxylic acid; HMG-CoA, 3-hydroxy-3-methylglutaryl-CoA; ETF, electron transfer flavoprotein.

patients who have frank metabolic acidosis with increased anion gaps would invariably miss patients affected with some of these disorders.

The clinical spectrum of the known disorders of organic acid metabolism spans a wide range of presentations involving almost every system in the body. In many cases, the urinary organic acid profile is typical of the disease, and diagnosis is relatively easy. In others, the abnormalities may be quite subtle, or only present intermittently. Table 4.5 presents disorders of organic acid metabolism organized according to the principal pathologic urinary organic acid abnormalities. The clinical aspects of many of the conditions listed are discussed in other parts of the book more appropriate to the nature of the clinical presentation.

Some of the conditions merit specific discussion either because they are relatively common, the interpretation of the clinical and laboratory findings may be difficult, or they serve to illustrate some general principle.

Methylmalonic acidemia (MMA)

MMA is a relatively common disorder of organic acid metabolism. However, the metabolism of methylmalonic acid is complex, involving the interaction of a number of distinct gene products and environmental factors (Figure 4.5). Deficiency or a defect in any one of them might produce methylmalonate accumulation. Classical methylmalonic acidemia is caused by complete deficiency of methylmalonyl-CoA mutase (mut), which normally catalyzes the rearrangement of methylmalonyl-CoA to succinyl-CoA. It commonly presents in the newborn period in a manner clinically indistinguishable from propionic acidemia (see Chapter 8) with severe metabolic acidosis, acute encephalopathy, hyperammonemia, neutropenia, and thrombocytopenia. Late-onset variants of the disease, in which residual mut activity is high, are common. Generally, the later the onset, the milder the disease; some individuals with methylmalonic acidemia as a result of mut mutations show no symptoms at all.

Methylmalonyl-CoA mutase is one of only two human enzymes known to require cobalamin (vitamin B_{12}) for activity. MMA caused by defects in the intramitochondrial processing or adenosylation of cobalamin (cblA and cblB variants, respectively), and defects affecting the affinity of mut for adenosylcobalamin, is often somewhat milder than disease caused by complete mut deficiency, and it is dramatically responsive to treatment with pharmacologic doses of vitamin B_{12}. In every other respects, it is clinically indistinguishable from classical MMA.

Methionine synthase (MS) is the other enzyme in the body which requires cobalamin for activity. In this case, the active form of the cofactor is methylcobalamin. Defects in the processing of MS-Cbl (cblE and cblG variants)

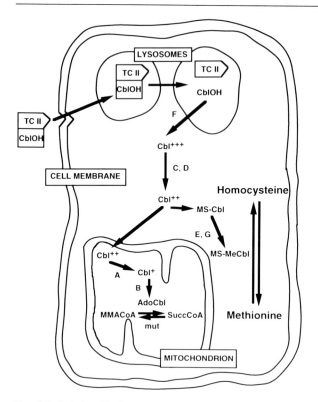

Fig. 4.5. Relationship between cobalamin, methylmalonic acid (MMA), and homocysteine metabolism.
The letters, A to F, refer to the locations of the metabolic defects of the different complementation groups of inherited defects in cobalamin metabolism.
Abbreviations: Cbl, cobalamin; TC II, transcobalamin II; MS-Cbl, methionine synthase-bound cobalamin; MMACoA, methylmalonyl-CoA; SuccCoA, succinyl-CoA; AdoCbl, adenosylcobalamin; mut, methylmalonyl-CoA mutase.

cause homocystinemia and homocystinuria, but not MMA. Patients with *cblE* and *cblG* disease present early in life with psychomotor retardation, feeding difficulties and failure to thrive, hypotonia, cerebral atrophy, and megaloblastic anemia that is hematologically indistinguishable from that caused by vitamin B_{12} deficiency. In contrast to the marked elevation of plasma methionine concentrations in classical homocystinuria due to cystathionine β-synthase deficiency, the methionine levels in patients with *cblE* and *cblG* defects are, as one would expect, decreased below normal.

Defects in the transport, intracellular uptake, lysosomal processing, release from lysosomes, or reduction of Cbl^{+++} to Cbl^{++} are characterized biochemically by both MMA and homocyst(e)inemia and homocystinuria. All these defects are associated with megaloblastic anemia, variable psychomotor retardation, and failure to thrive, some with onset in early infancy and others only emerging in later life. Patients with hereditary defects in cobalamin processing (*cblC*, *cblD*, and *cblF* variants) generally have more severe disease than those with defects in cobalamin absorption and transport (e.g., *transcobalamin II deficiency*). Developmental retardation, failure to thrive, seizures, and megaloblastic anemia are prominent, along with MMA and homocystinuria. Although symptoms of feeding difficulty and hypotonia often develop in the first few weeks of life (especially in *cblC* disease), urinary methylmalonic acid levels are never as high as in MMA due to mut deficiency, and acute metabolic acidosis with hyperammonemia does not occur, even in patients with early-onset variants of these cobalamin defects. The clinical variability among patients with different cobalamin defects is considerable making classification of the defects on clinical grounds alone unreliable. As a rule, definitive classification requires complementation studies on cultured skin fibroblasts (see Chapter 9).

Over the years, we have encountered a number of infants presenting in the first few months of life with MMA, megaloblastic anemia, and homocystinuria with normal or low plasma methionine levels, as a result of dietary vitamin B$_{12}$ deficiency. In every case, the mother was a strict vegan and the infant was breast fed. The cause of the metabolic abnormalities in each case was confirmed by demonstrating that plasma vitamin B$_{12}$ levels were well below normal.

3-Hydroxy-3-methylglutaryl-CoA (HMG-CoA) lyase deficiency

HMG-CoA lyase catalyzes the last step in the intramitochondrial catabolism of the amino acid, leucine (Figure 4.4). The products of the reaction, acetoacetate and acetyl-CoA, are important energy substrates, particularly during illness or fasting. Patients with HMG-CoA lyase deficiency may present in the newborn period, in a manner resembling neonatal propionic acidemia or MMA, with severe metabolic acidosis, vomiting, lethargy and drowsiness progressing to coma, poor feeding, hypoglycemia in most, and hyperammonemia in many. However, HMG-CoA lyase deficiency is different from the other organic acidopathies presenting with similar symptoms because of the absence of ketonuria. The disease presenting for the first time in older infants often resembles Reye syndrome or a fatty acid oxidation defect, such as medium-chain acyl-CoA dehydrogenase (MCAD) deficiency (see Chapter 2). The findings of enlargement of the liver and abnormal liver function tests add to the potential for diagnostic confusion. However, urinary organic acid analysis characteristically shows abnormalities typical of the disease, particularly during metabolic crises: massive excretion of 3-hydroxy-3-methylglutarate and 3-methylglutaconate, and large amounts of 3-hydroxyisovalerate, 3-methylglutarate. Lactic acidosis and marked increases in urinary glutaric acid and adipic acid levels are often seen during very severe metabolic crises. Plasma carnitine levels are decreased and the proportion of esterified carnitine is increased as a result of the formation of 3-methylglutarylcarnitine; neither HMG or 3-methylglutaconate form carnitine esters in patients with this disease. Treatment is effective in decreasing the frequency and severity of episodes of acute metabolic decompensation. In spite of apparently adequate treatment, with a high carbohydrate, low protein diet supplemented with carnitine, some patients develop cardiomyopathy which may be fatal.

Glutaric aciduria

Glutaric aciduria type I (GA I), caused by deficiency of mitochondrial glutaryl-CoA dehydrogenase, usually presents in early infancy as a neurologic syndrome (see Chapter 2). After some weeks or months of apparently normal development, affected infants suddenly develop the first of recurrent episodes of marked hypotonia, dystonia, opisthotonus, grimacing, fisting, tongue thrusting, and seizures. Partial recovery is followed by progressive neurologic deterioration and periodic episodes of ketoacidosis, vomiting, and acute encephalopathy resembling Reye syndrome, usually precipitated by intercurrent infections. In some patients, the neurologic abnormalities remain relatively stationary with gross motor retardation, chronic choreoathetosis, dystonia, and hypotonia, with apparent preservation of intellect. CNS imaging studies show early cortical atrophy and attenuation of white matter and basal ganglia. Some patients present with acute Reye-like disease without the extrapyramidal neurologic signs. During acute metabolic decompensation, laboratory studies show metabolic acidosis and ketosis, hypoglycemia, hyperammonemia, and mild hepatocellular dysfunction. Besides marked increases in glutaric acid concentration, urinary organic acid analysis shows the the presence of 3-hydroxyglutarate, considered pathognomonic of the disease, and sometimes glutaconic acid during severe ketoacidosis. Between episodes of metabolic decompensation, the urinary organic acids may be normal or only mildly abnormal. Plasma carnitine levels are decreased.

Glutaric aciduria type II (GA II), which is also called multiple acyl-CoA dehydrogenase deficiency, is caused by deficiency of either electron transport flavoprotein (ETF) or ETF dehydrogenase, the intramitochondrial electron-

Table 4.6. *Flavoprotein dehydrogenases for which*
ETF/ETF dehydrogenase is the electron acceptor.

Mitochondrial fatty acid β-oxidation
Very long-chain acyl-CoA dehydrogenase
Long-chain acyl-CoA (LCAD) dehydrogenase
Medium-chain acyl-CoA (MCAD) dehydrogenase
Short-chain acyl-CoA (SCAD) dehydrogenase

Leucine oxidation
Isovaleryl-CoA dehydrogenase

Valine and isoleucine oxidation
2-Methylbutyryl-CoA dehydrogenase

Lysine, hydroxylysine, and tryptophan oxidation
Glutaryl-CoA dehydrogenase

Choline oxidation
Dimethylglycine dehydrogenase
Sarcosine dehydrogenase

Note: Abbreviation: ETF, electron transfer flavoprotein.

acceptors for a number of acyl-CoA dehydrogenases (Table 4.6). The condition may present in one of three ways:

- Very severe, neonatal disease, characterized by facial dysmorphism, muscular defects of the abdominal wall, hypospadias (in males), cystic disease of the kidneys, hypotonia, hepatomegaly, hypoketotic hypoglycemia, metabolic acidosis, and hyperammonemia (see Chapter 8).
- Severe neonatal disease without dysmorphism, but with hypotonia, hepatomegaly, hypoketotic hypoglycemia, metabolic acidosis, and hyperammonemia.
- Mild disease characterized by later-onset episodic acute metabolic acidosis, failure to thrive, hypoglycemia, hyperammonemia, and encephalopathy.

The severe variants are often associated with a peculiar odor of sweaty feet similar to that seen in infants with severe isovaleric acidemia. Plasma amino acid analysis shows elevations of several amino acids, especially proline and hydroxyproline. Urinary organic acid analysis in infants with severe variants of the disease characteristically shows very large amounts of glutarate, ethylmalonate, and the dicarboxylic acids, adipate, suberate, and sebacate, in addition to isovalerate, isovalerylglycine, 2-hydroxyglutarate, hexanoylglycine, and 5-hydroxyhexanoate. The mild form of GA II is often called ethylmalonic-adipic aciduria, referring to the predominant urinary organic acid abnormalities. However, the urinary organic acids may be normal between episodes of metabolic decompensation.

Secondary glutaric aciduria is much more common than glutaric aciduria due to primary disorders of glutaric acid metabolism, like GA I and GA II. It is commonly found in relatively large concentrations in infants with mitochondrial ETC defects, presumably a reflection of 'sick mitochondria'. We have also seen massive glutaric aciduria in a boy with late-onset, but severely decompensated propionic acidemia. It has been reported in 2-ketoadipic acidemia (α-aminoadipic acidemia), probably as a result of nonenzymic decarboxylation of 2-ketoadipate. It is also one of the dicarboxylic acids appearing in the urine of infants on medium-chain triglyceride formulas.

Dicarboxylic aciduria

Increased concentration of the medium-chain dicarboxylic acids, adipic (6-carbon), suberic (8-carbon), and sebacic (10-carbon) acids, is one of the most prominent laboratory abnormalities in patients with inherited disorders of mitochondrial fatty acid β-oxidation, such as medium-chain acyl-CoA dehydrogenase (MCAD) deficiency. These disorders usually present as acute neurologic or hepatic syndromes, rather than as metabolic acidosis (see Chapters 2 and 5).

Medium-chain dicarboxylic aciduria is also a common secondary feature of several other conditions. The levels of adipic, suberic, and sebacic acids in the urine are generally increased under any circumstances in which fatty acid utilization is increased beyond the capacity for mitochondrial β-oxidation, such as during starvation and in patients with diabetes mellitus. It is also commonly seen in patients on the anticonvulsant, valproic acid, which inhibits fatty acid β-oxidation, and in newborn infants. When the dicarboxylic aciduria is the result of increased fatty acid oxidation, it is routinely associated with marked ketosis and the excretion of large amounts of 3-hydroxybutyrate (3-HOB) and acetoacetate. The ratio of 3-HOB to adipate is generally $>0.5–1.0$. By contrast, in patients with mitochondrial fatty acid β-oxidation defects, the urinary ketone concentrations are characteristically low, and the 3-HOB/adipate ratio is <1.0. Unfortunately, in very young infants, or in infants on formulas containing medium-chain triglycerides, the relationship breaks down; many apparently healthy newborn infants, particularly low birth-weight premature infants, excrete amounts of medium chain dicarboxylic acids comparable to the levels seen in asymptomatic infants with fatty acid oxidation defects. Analyses of urinary acylglycines and acylcarnitines, and especially measurements of plasma acylcarnitines, are particularly helpful in distinguishing infants with genetic defects in fatty acid metabolism.

Ethylmalonic aciduria

Ethylmalonate and adipate are particularly prominent in the urine of patients with the mild variant of multiple acyl-CoA dehydrogenase deficiency (GA II). However, ethylmalonate is excreted in a wide variety of other circumstances, some associated with severe systemic inherited metabolic diseases, others being quite benign.

Increased concentrations of ethylmalonate, along with methylsuccinate, may be the only urinary organic abnormalities in the urine of patients with short-chain acyl-CoA dehydrogenase (SCAD) deficiency. Ethylmalonic aciduria, without methylsuccinate, is also found in patients with cytochrome c oxidase deficiency. The combination of lactic acidosis, ethylmalonic, and methylsuccinic aciduria, along with the excretion of butyrylglycine, isovalerylglycine, and 2-methylbutyrylglycine, is characteristic of a condition characterized clinically by severe psychomotor retardation, spasticity, chronic diarrhea, and orthostatic acrocyanosis. The underlying metabolic defect in affected infants is still not known, though defects in 2-methylbranched chain acyl-CoA dehydrogenase or cytochrome c oxidase have been suggested.

D-Lactic acidosis

Infants or young children with gastrointestinal abnormalities, such as blind loops, involving bowel stasis, sometimes develop attacks of severe metabolic acidosis, often associated with acute encephalopathy, with increased anion gap. Plasma lactate, 3-hydroxybutyrate, and acetoacetate levels may be completely normal. However, organic acid analysis shows the presence of large amounts of lactic acid in the urine. The acidosis in these cases is not the result of an inborn error of metabolism; it is caused by accumulation of D-lactate, a product of bacterial carbohydrate metabolism which is readily absorbed from the gut. The routine measurement of lactate in blood is by an enzymic method, employing LDH, which is specific for L-lactate, the usual product of carbohydrate metabolism in humans. Urinary organic acid analysis is generally carried out by chromatographic techniques, such as gas chromatography-mass spectrometry (GC-MS), which do not differentiate the D-isomer of lactate from the L-isomer. The marked discrepancy between the results of lactate measurements by the two techniques provides the clue to the origin of the acidosis. Treatment with antimicrobials usually produces rapid resolution of the acidosis, though recurrence of the problem is common.

Table 4.7. *Some common causes of spurious or artefactual organic aciduria.*

Organic acid	Underlying condition or disease
D-Lactic acid	Intestinal bacterial over-growth. May be sufficient to cause metabolic acidosis and encephalopathy.
Methylmalonic, ethylmalonic, and 3-hydroxypropionic acids	Very young infants with gastroenteritis; may be associated with methemoglobinemia.
Medium-chain dicarboxylic acids (adipic acid > suberic > sebacic)	Valproic acid administration. The pattern often resembles that seen in patients with defects in mitochondrial fatty acid oxidation.
Medium-chain dicarboxylic acids (sebacic > suberic > adipic)	Ingestion of formulas containing medium-chain triglycerides. The relationship between the organic acids varies according to the fatty acid composition of the medium chain triglyceride.
Adipic acid	Ingestion of large amounts of Jello® containing adipic acid additive. The elevation of adipate may be large, but the absence of any other organic acid abnormality suggests the underlying dietary etiology.
Long-chain 3-hydroxydicarboxylic acids	Acetaminophen intoxication; severe hepatocellular disease.
Pivalic acid (5-carbon acylcarnitine may be indistinguishable from isovalerylcarnitine)	Pivampicillin or pivmecillinam administration.
Octenylsuccinic acid	Formulas containing octenylsuccinate-modified cornstarch as emulsifying agent.
Methylmalonic acid	A prominent feature of vitamin B_{12} deficiency.
Azelaic and pimelic acids	Extracts from plastic storage containers.
2-Hydroxybutyric acid	Occurs with severe lactic acidosis, irrespective of the cause.
5-Oxoproline (pyroglutamic acid)	Acetaminophen or vigabatrin ingestion.

Adventitious organic aciduria

In addition to expanding tremendously the number of identified inherited metabolic diseases, the widespread application of urinary organic analysis has also posed some challenging problems in interpretation owing to the effects of age, bowel flora, intercurrent illness, and medications, on urinary organic acid excretion. Some of the more common causes of urinary organic acid artifacts are shown in Table 4.7.

Bibliography

Goldstein, M.B., Bear, R., Richardson, R.M.A., Marsden, P.A. & Halperin, M.L. (1986). The urine anion gap: a clinically useful index of ammonium excretion. *American Journal of Medical Science*, **292**, 198–202.

Kohlschuter, A. (1983). The clinical presentation of organicacidopathies – when to investigate. *Neuropediatrics*, **14**, 191–6.

Lehotay, D. & Clarke, J. T. R. (1995). Organic acidurias and related abnormalities. *Critical Reviews in Clinical Laboratory Sciences*, **32**, 377–429.

Mitchell, G.A., Kassovska-Bratinova, S., Boukaftane, Y., Robert, M.-F., Wang, S.P., Ashmarina, L., Lambert, M., LaPierre, P. & Potier, E. (1995). Medical aspects of ketone body metabolism. *Clinical and Investigative Medicine*, **18**, 193–216.

Ozand, P.T. & Gascon, G.G. (1991). Organic acidurias: a review, Parts 1 and 2. *Journal of Child Neurology*, **6**, 196–219 and 288–303.

Rabier, D., Bardet, J., Parvy, Ph., Poggi, F., Brivet, M., Saudubray, J.M. & Kamoun, P. (1995). Do criteria exist from urinary organic acids to distinguish β-oxidation defects? *Journal of Inherited Metabolic Diseases*, **18**, 257–60.

Robinson, B.H. (1993). Lacticacidemia. *Biochimica et Biophysica Acta*, **1182**, 231–44.

Stacpoole, P.W. (1993). Lactic acidosis. *Endocrinology and Metabolism Clinics of North America*, **22**, 221–45.

Winters, R.W. (1982). *Principles of Pediatric Fluid Therapy*, 2nd edn. Boston: Little, Brown and Company.

5

Hepatic syndrome

Liver involvement of some kind is a presenting feature of a number of inherited metabolic diseases. The metabolic activities of the liver span a vast catalogue of functions important to the metabolism of the entire body. It is surprising, therefore, that the repertoire of responses to injury is limited, and inborn errors of metabolism manifesting as hepatic syndrome are commonly difficult to distinguish from many acquired conditions, such as infections, intoxications, developmental abnormalities, and neoplasia. One approach to the diagnosis of inherited metabolic diseases presenting as hepatic syndrome is to consider four possible presentations, recognizing that there is considerable overlap between them. They are:

- jaundice;
- hepatomegaly;
- hypoglycemia;
- hepatocellular dysfunction.

Jaundice
Jaundice is caused by accumulation of unconjugated or conjugated bilirubin, which may occur as a result of increased production, impaired metabolism, or biliary obstruction. Bilirubin is a porphyrin pigment derived from the degradative metabolism of the heme of hemoglobin.

Unconjugated hyperbilirubinemia
Pure unconjugated hyperbilirubinemia is characteristic of disorders associated with increased bilirubin production. Mature erythrocytes have no mitochondria. They derive virtually all the energy needed to maintain ion gradients, intracellular nucleotide concentrations, membrane plasticity, the iron of hemoglobin in the reduced state, and other functions, from glycolysis and activity of the hexose monophosphate shunt. Not surprisingly, specific hereditary deficiencies of any

of the enzymes involved commonly present with hemolytic anemia. Some are also associated with neurologic symptoms, such as severe psychomotor retardation (e.g., triosephosphate isomerase deficiency) or myopathy (e.g., phosphofructokinase deficiency) (see Chapter 2). The hyperbilirubinemia caused by hemolysis is characteristically unconjugated, and it is not generally accompanied by any clinical or biochemical evidence of hepatocellular dysfunction.

The commonest inborn error of erythrocyte metabolism presenting as jaundice is X-linked recessive *glucose-6-phosphate dehydrogenase* (G6PD) *deficiency*, a defect in the first reaction of the hexose monophosphate shunt. Carriers of the gene show relative resistance to malaria accounting for the high prevalence of the mutation in areas of the world, such as central Africa, where it is endemic. Acute hemolysis is typically precipitated by intercurrent illness or exposure to oxidizing drugs, such as certain sulfonamides and certain antimalarials, though it may occur spontaneously in the newborn period. The commonest inborn error of glycolysis presenting as unconjugated hyperbilirubinemia is *pyruvate kinase* (PK) *deficiency* which, like G6PD deficiency, may present in the newborn period with severe nonspherocytic hemolytic anemia.

Unconjugated hyperbilirubinemia is also a feature of some primary disorders of bilirubin metabolism. Normal bilirubin metabolism involves uptake by hepatocytes, conjugation with glucuronic acid, and excretion in bile. At least some individuals with *Gilbert syndrome*, a common (3% of the population), benign disorder of bilirubin metabolism associated with mild persistent unconjugated hyperbilirubinemia, generally presenting after puberty, appear to have a defect in bilirubin uptake along with partial deficiency of bilirubin UDP-glucuronosyltransferase (BGT). The absence of any evidence of hemolysis or hepatocellular dysfunction is typical of individuals with this condition.

Severe neonatal unconjugated hyperbilirubinemia caused by specific BGT deficiency is characteristic of *Crigler-Najjar syndrome*. It is commonly associated with unconjugated bilirubin levels > 500 μmol/L in the absence of any evidence of hemolysis, infection, or significant hepatocellular dysfunction. Phototherapy and exchange transfusion are ineffective, and affected infants invariably develop severe kernicterus. Some patients, classified as Crigler-Najjar syndrome type 2 (also called *Arias syndrome*), respond to administration of phenobarbital (4 mg/kg/day) with a dramatic drop in plasma bilirubin levels. Patients with Crigler-Najjar syndrome are not usually difficult to distinguish from patients with breast milk jaundice, which is milder, later in onset, and can be shown to be associated with breast-feeding.

It is important to remember that the hyperbilirubinemia in infants with *classical galactosemia* is often initially unconjugated, converting only after a period of some days to the conjugated hyperbilirubinemia widely regarded as characteristic of the disease. Even early in the course of the disease, galactosemia is associated with evidence of significant hepatocellular dysfunction which sets it apart from Crigler-Najjar syndrome. Galactosemia is discussed in more detail in the section 'Hepatocellular dysfunction'.

Conjugated hyperbilirubinemia
Conjugated hyperbilirubinemia as a manifestation of inherited metabolic disease is more common than unconjugated hyperbilirubinemia because it includes those diseases, like galactosemia, hepatorenal tyrosinemia, and hereditary fructose intolerance, in which hepatocellular dysfunction is prominent (see 'Hepatocellular dysfunction'). Mixed conjugated and unconjugated hyper-bilirubinemia in the absence of any other evidence of hepatocellular dysfunction or hemolysis, with onset in later childhood, is typical of patients with *Rotor syndrome* or *Dubin-Johnson syndrome* caused by benign defects in the intrahepatic biliary excretion of bilirubin glucuronide. The two conditions are differentiated from each other by differences in urinary porphyrins. The former is associated with a marked increase in urinary excretion of coproporphyrin I and III with < 80% being the I isomer; in Dubin-Johnson syndrome, the urinary coproporphyrin levels may be normal, but the I isomer accounts for > 80% of the total (normal about 25%).

Hepatomegaly
Asymptomatic hepatomegaly is common in children, and the decision about who to investigate, and how intensively, is sometimes difficult. The hepatomegaly associated with inherited metabolic diseases is generally persistent and nontender. If the liver is so soft that the edge is difficult to palpate, enlargement is likely to be due to accumulation of triglyceride, a typical feature of GSD (glycogen storage disease) type I. At the other extreme, a hard and irregular liver edge, often associated with only modest enlargement of the organ, is characteristic of cirrhosis, such as is characteristic of *hepatorenal tyrosinemia* (hereditary tyrosinemia, type I). When it is enlarged as a result of lysosomal storage, the liver is usually firm, but not hard.

Is the spleen also enlarged? A history of hematemesis or the presence of ascites, or abdominal venous dilatation, would suggest that splenomegaly is caused by portal hypertension resulting from cirrhosis. However, the spleen may be enlarged by infiltration or accumulation of the same cells or metabolites causing enlargement of the liver. Besides sharing the portal circulation, the liver and spleen both contain components of the reticuloendothelial system (RES). Conditions causing expansion of the RES, either as a result of cellular proliferation or storage within RES cells (i.e., macrophages), commonly present with clinical enlargement of both organs. This is characteristic, for example, of many of the lysosomal storage diseases.

Glycogen storage disease, type III, (GSD III) commonly presents as asymptomatic hepatomegaly discovered incidentally in the course of routine physical examination. The spleen may also be enlarged, but the splenomegaly is mild compared with the enlargement of the liver. Glycogen accumulation in this condition is caused by deficiency of a debrancher enzyme which converts the branch-points in glycogen into linear molecules for further hydrolysis by phosphorylase. The enlargement of the liver may be marked. It is generally firm and nontender, with a sharp, smooth, edge which is easy to palpate. In most patients, hypoglycemia does not occur, or it occurs only after prolonged fasting. However, in a significant minority, it may present in early infancy and be as severe as the hypoglycemia seen in patients with GSD I. Severe early infantile GSD III may also be associated with failure to thrive and hyperlipidemia, further blurring the clinical differentiation from GSD I. However, lactic acidosis and hyperuricemia do not occur, or are very mild, in patients with GSD III. Moreover, the condition is associated with ketosis during fasting and with moderate increases in liver aminotransferases (AST and ALT), which, as a rule, do not occur in GSD I. Liver biospy shows increased glycogen with variable interlobular fibrosis, but very little fat. Rarely, the fibrosis progresses to frank cirrhosis producing portal hypertension and liver failure. As adults, many affected patients develop evidence of muscle involvement, including cardiomyopathy in some. This is characterized by proximal muscle weakness, depressed deep tendon reflexes, and elevation of plasma creatine phosphokinase (see Chapter 2).

Patients with GSD III will show a rise in plasma glucose in response to ingestion of galactose, fructose, or amino acids, indicating that gluconeogenesis is intact. They also show a significant increase in plasma glucose in response to glucagon administered two to four hours after feeding, but they do not respond after 10–12 hours of fasting when all the hepatic linear glycogen accessible to phosphorylase activity has been depleted. Confirmation of the diagnosis requires measurement of debrancher enzyme activity in fresh liver obtained by biopsy.

Hepatic phosphorylase deficiency (GSD VI) is often clinically indistinguishable from GSD III, though it is much less common, and involvement of skeletal muscle and the heart does not occur. Phosphorylase deficiency can be demonstrated histochemically on tissue obtained by biopsy.

Phosphorylase b *kinase deficiency* is more common than GSD VI. The most common variant appears to be transmitted as an X-linked recessive disorder.

Clinically, it is often indistinguishable from GSD III. However, unlike patients with GSD III, patients with phosphorylase *b* kinase deficiency show only minimal increases in plasma glucose in response to glucagon after fasting of any duration. Liver biopsy shows increased glycogen, which may be more dispersed in appearance than in GSD III. There is often some interlobular fibrosis, though cirrhosis is rare. Confirmation of the diagnosis is best done by direct enzyme analysis of fresh liver, although some patients show deficiency of the enzyme in red blood cells. Involvement of skeletal muscle occurs in a small proportion of patients, in whom the condition appears to be transmitted as an autosomal recessive. Isolated involvement of skeletal muscle or the myocardium is very rare (see Chapters 2 and 6).

Hypoglycemia

Hunger, apprehension, jitters, irritability, and sweating are common early symptoms of hypoglycemia in older patients. Unless the cause of the symptoms is recognized and treated, this is followed by disturbance of consciousness with drowsiness progressing rapidly to stupor and coma accompanied by convulsions. Idiosyncratic presentations dominated by behavioural abnormalities are common. In very young infants, the early signs may be subtle with nothing more than irritability, sweating, and somnolence. A seizure may be the first recognized indication of the problem, and hypoglycemia should be considered in any infant presenting for the first time with convulsions. Treatment with intravenous glucose should not be delayed.

The differential diagnosis of hypoglycemia is made easier by some understanding of the normal mechanisms for maintaining normal plasma glucose concentrations during fasting. During the intervals between meals, the plasma glucose concentration is supported by two general mechanisms:

- mechanisms directed at producing glucose (glycogen breakdown and gluconeogenesis);
- mechanisms which decrease peripheral glucose utilization by providing alternative energy substrates (fatty acid and ketone oxidation).

Hypoglycemia may occur as a result of primary or secondary defects in glucose production (deficiency of supply), or as a result of defects in fatty acid or ketone oxidation (over-utilization).

Ways to increase glucose production

Glycogen is a high-molecular weight, highly branched polymer of glucose. During feeding it is formed by polymerization of glucose, derived primarily from

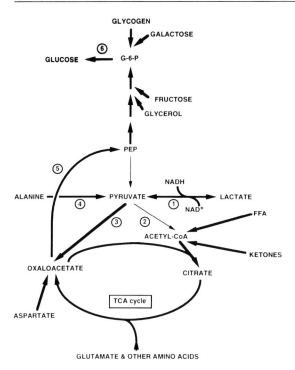

Fig. 5.1. Overview of key reactions in gluconeogenesis.
The various enzymes involved in key reactions of gluconeogenesis are: **1**, lactate dehydrogenase (LDH); **2**, pyruvate dehydrogenase complex (PDH); **3**, pyruvate carboxylase (PC); **4**, alanine aminotransferase (ALT); **5**, phosphoenolpyruvate carboxykinase (PEPCK); **6**, glucose-6-phosphatase.

dietary carbohydrate. During fasting, the process is reversed with glucose being released by phosphorylase-catalyzed hydrolysis of glycogen. Glycogen is an excellent form of immediately available glucose. However, storage in the liver involves the simultaneous storage of large amounts of water, and the total amount of glycogen that can be accommodated in the space available in the liver is, therefore, actually relatively small. As a result, within only 24–48 hours of fasting, the glycogen in the liver becomes totally depleted as it is rapidly converted into glucose to meet the immediate needs of tissues, like the brain, having high energy requirements.

The synthesis of glucose from nonglucose substrates (gluconeogenesis) occurs coincidentally with glycogenolysis during fasting, and it is ultimately capable of supplying much more glucose over a longer period of time. The process (Figure 5.1), which takes place predominantly in the cytosol, is functionally the reverse of glycolysis. One of the most important regulatory steps in the process is the carboxylation of pyruvate to form oxaloacetate (catalyzed by pyruvate carboxylase) within mitochondria. The oxaloacetate formed by the reaction is then converted to phosphoenolpyruvate in a reaction catalyzed by mitochondrial phosphoenolpyruvate carboxykinase (PEPCK). The PEP diffuses out of the mitochondria into the cytoplasm where it is converted to glucose in a series of reactions which mirror the same steps in glycolysis.

Oxaloacetate is also transported out of mitochondria into the cytoplasm by the 'malate shuttle'. Cytosolic oxaloacetate is converted to PEP by cytosolic PEPCK, which is genetically distinct from the mitochondrial isozyme. There is some evidence that mitochondrial PEPCK is particularly important in the synthesis of glucose from pyruvate derived from lactate, and that cytosolic PEPCK is more important in gluconeogenesis involving oxaloacetate and pyruvate derived from amino acid metabolism.

Other important gluconeogenic substrates, such as galactose, fructose, and glycerol, feed into the process at different steps between PEP and glucose-6-phosphate. The final step in *both* glycogenolysis and gluconeogenesis is glucose-6-phosphatase-catalyzed hydrolysis of glucose-6-phosphate to form free glucose.

A critical aspect of gluconeogenesis is an adjustment made to preserve and re-utilize the carbon skeleton of glucose, rather than having it lost irretrievably as a result of oxidation all the way to CO_2. This process, which is called the Cori cycle (Figure 5.2), involves the simultaneous synthesis of glucose from pyruvate in the liver (gluconeogenesis) and partial oxidation of glucose to pyruvate (glycolysis) in the periphery, primarily in muscle. The partial oxidation of glucose by glycolysis yields only a fraction of the ATP that could be derived from total oxidation to CO_2 and water. However, the capacity to re-synthesize glucose, using energy derived largely from fatty acid oxidation, more than compensates for the inefficiency: the trade-off is expanded capacity in exchange for decreased efficiency.

Ways to decrease peripheral glucose utilization
The capacity to derive energy from mitochondrial fatty acid β-oxidation is a critically important mechanism for sparing glucose. The storage efficiency of energy as triglyceride is much greater than as hepatic glycogen. Long after liver glycogen has been depleted by starvation, the body continues to draw on the triglyceride in adipose tissue to provide an alternative to glucose for energy production. The process decreases the need for glucose production to a minimum, sparing it for various biosynthetic processes and for use by tissues, like

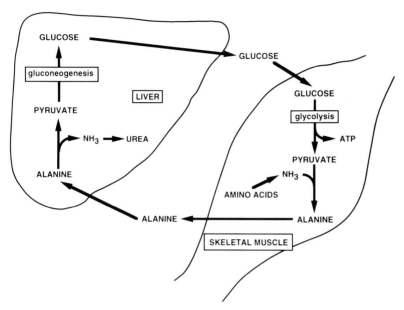

Fig. 5.2. The Cori cycle.

red blood cells, which cannot meet their energy needs any other way. Organs, like the brain, which do not derive significant amounts of energy from fatty acid β-oxidation within the tissue itself, oxidize ketones produced by fatty acid oxidation in the liver. The relationship between hepatic ketogenesis and peripheral ketone utilization is reviewed in Chapter 4.

During starvation, increased secretion of epinephrine and glucagon stimulates hormone-sensitive lipase in adipose tissue to break down triglyceride into free fatty acids and glycerol. The glycerol is taken up by the liver and converted into glucose by gluconeogenesis (Figure 5.1). The fatty acids are transported in the circulation bound to albumin to tissues like liver and muscle where they are taken up, activated by esterification with coenzyme A, and transported into mitochondria, by a process dependent on availability of carnitine. In mitochondria, they undergo β-oxidation with the production of energy in the form of ATP. In the liver, the principal intermediate in the process, acetyl-CoA, is converted to ketones (3-hydroxybutyrate and acetoacetate) for export via the circulation to tissues, such as the brain, able to regenerate acetyl-CoA, and complete the oxidation of the compound to produce ATP. Defects in ketone utilization are characterized by intermittent, severe ketoacidosis (see Chapter 4).

Free fatty acids and their coenzyme A esters are toxic. When the mobilization

Table 5.1. *Causes of secondary carnitine deficiency.*

Decreased biosynthesis
Chronic liver disease
Chronic renal disease
Extreme prematurity

Inadequate intake (nutritional)
Prolonged TPN in premature infants
Severe protein calorie malnutrition
Intestinal malabsorption
Vegetarian diet

Increased losses
Renal tubular dysfunction
Renal failure (uremia)
Hemodialysis
Organic acidopathies (PA, MMA, etc.)
Treatment with valproic acid
UCED treated with long-term sodium benzoate

Note: Abbreviations: TPN, total parenteral nutrition; UCED, urea cycle enzyme defects; PA, propionic acidemia; MMA, methylmalonic acidemia.
Source: See Pons & De Vivo (1995).

of fatty acids is increased, or the capacity for mitochondrial β-oxidation is exceeded, for whatever reason, any excess fatty acid is converted back to triglyceride, or it is oxidized by nonmitochondrial systems, such as microsomal ω-oxidation and peroxisomal β-oxidation (see Figure 5.5). Mitochondrial fatty acid β-oxidation depends critically on the availability of adequate amounts of carnitine. Although carnitine is synthesized endogenously, and generally occurs in ample quantities in the diet, secondary deficiency is quite common (Table 5.1). No primary disorder of carnitine biosynthesis has ever been found. However, carnitine deficiency does occur as a result of genetic defects in its cellular transport. This may take the form of systemic carnitine deficiency, characterized clinically by recurrent attacks of Reye-like encephalopathy with hypoketotic hypoglycemia or severe cardiomyopathy. Skeletal myopathy also occurs in patients with transport defects, apparently limited to the uptake of carnitine by muscle.

Carnitine also provides an alternative to coenzyme A (CoASH) in the esterification of organic acid intermediates of amino acid metabolism. Exchanging the coenzyme A of organic acyl-CoA esters with carnitine frees CoASH. CoASH is required by many processes in intermediary metabolism, particularly related to gluconeogenesis and ammonium metabolism. In patients with inborn errors of organic acid metabolism, such as methylmalonic acidemia, acylcarnitine esters accumulate and are excreted in the urine causing secondary carnitine depletion.

Within the mitochondrial matrix, fatty acyl-CoA undergoes β-oxidation. The process involves four enzymic steps operating in a cycle to shorten a fatty acyl-CoA chain by two carbons with the release of one molecule of acetyl-CoA per turn (see Figure 9.5). Several of the steps in fatty acid transport and oxidation are catalyzed by different enzymes having different substrate chain-length specificities. The most important of these from the standpoint of inherited disorders of fatty acid oxidation, is the first step, catalyzed by four different fatty acyl-CoA dehydrogenase enzymes: very long-chain acyl-CoA dehydrogenase (VLCAD), long-chain acyl-CoA dehydrogenase (LCAD), medium-chain acyl-CoA dehydrogenase (MCAD), and short-chain acyl-CoA dehydrogenase (SCAD).

The electrons derived from the various fatty acyl-CoA dehydrogenase reactions are transferred to a common electron transport flavoprotein (ETF) which is oxidized in turn by a reaction catalyzed by ETF dehydrogenase. ETF dehydrogenase catalyzes the transfer of electrons to Coenzyme Q, part of Complex II of the mitochondrial electron transport chain (see Figure 9.7). Mutations affecting the amount or function of ETF or ETF dehydrogenase cause multiple acyl-CoA dehydrogenase deficiency (GA II). (See also Chapters 4 and 7.)

An approach to the differential diagnosis of hypoglycemia

Hypoglycemia is a common, nonspecific problem in severely ill neonates and young infants, regardless of the cause of the illness. Sometimes, whether the hypoglycemia is the cause, or a nonspecific result, of illness can be difficult at first to determine. Regardless of the cause, correction of hypoglycemia without delay is at least as important as making a specific diagnosis. As a rule, the hypoglycemia associated with severe systemic disease, such as sepsis, is relatively easy to control by administration of glucose at a rate at, or slightly greater than, the normal basal glucose oxidation rate (4–6 mg/kg/min in neonates and 3–5 mg/kg/min in older infants and children). Figure 5.3 shows an overview of one approach to the diagnosis of hypoglycemia, focusing primarily on that caused by inborn errors of metabolism.

The presence of nonglucose reducing substances in the urine is characteristic of untreated classical galactosemia and hereditary fructose intolerance (HFI).

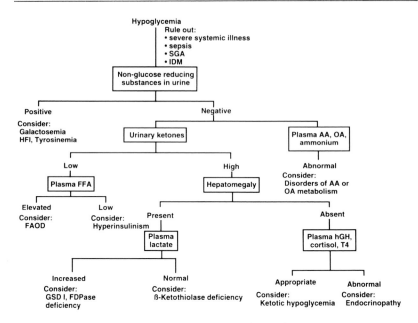

Fig. 5.3. Approach to the differential diagnosis of hypoglycemia.
Abbreviations: SGA, small for gestational age; IDM, infant of diabetic mother; HFI, hereditary fructose intolerance; AA, amino acids; OA, organic acids; FFA, free fatty acids; FAOD, fatty acid oxidation defect; hGH, human growth hormone; T4, thyroxine; GSD, glycogen storage disease; FDPase, fructose-,6-diphosphatase.

This is simple to determine at the bedside. Testing a few drops of urine with Benedict's reagent or with Clinitest tablets is positive in the presence of glucose, galactose, or fructose. However, dipping the same urine with Clinistix is usually negative in these conditions, indicating that the reducing substance is not glucose. Both diseases are generally associated with other prominent clinical problems. As a rule, patients with galactosemia have other evidence of hepatocellular dysfunction, and HFI is associated with marked lactic acidosis. The glycosuria in these conditions typically clears rapidly after removal of the toxic sugars from the diet. Therefore, a negative test does not eliminate the possibility of one of these disorders, particularly if the patient has been on intravenous glucose for more than a few hours.

Because hypoglycemia is a common secondary metabolic consequence of various inborn errors of amino acid and organic acid metabolism, the investigation of hypoglycemia should include analysis of urinary organic acids, and plasma amino acids and ammonium.

Primary defects in glucose production

The normal physiologic response to decreased glucose production is increased mitochondrial fatty acid β-oxidation and the production of ketones. Accordingly, urinary tests for ketones, another bedside test, provide an indirect indication of whether hypoglycemia is the result of inadequate production or of over-utilization of glucose. The hypoglycemia caused by insulin-induced over-utilization of glucose is characteristically associated with very low plasma and urine ketone concentrations (hypoketotic hypoglycemia). However, in some disorders of glucose production, such as GSD I and PEPCK deficiency, ketogenesis is often suppressed, and plasma and urinary ketone levels, though elevated, may be inappropriately low for the degree of hypoglycemia. The history of the relationship of the hypoglycemia to feeding is often helpful here. On the one hand, hypoketotic hypoglycemia developing within several minutes of feeding, particularly if it is severe, is typical of hyperinsulinism. On the other hand, patients with defects in glycogen breakdown, gluconeogensis, or fatty acid oxidation tend to tolerate short-term fasting much better. A significant exception is GSD I, and rare cases of GSD III, in which hypoglycemia may develop within two to three hours of feeding.

GSD I may present with hypoglycemia in the newborn period. However, it is typically not difficult to control and the liver may not be particularly enlarged. In fact, a normal three-hourly feeding schedule is generally sufficient to suppress symptomatic hypoglycemia. Affected infants usually come to attention at three to five months of age when prolonging the interval between feeds, or associated intercurrent illness, precipitates an episode of severe hypoglycemia, often heralded by a seizure or coma. Some infants come to attention as a result of failure to thrive, others because of massive hepatomegaly discovered incidentally during physical examination. Occasionally, an infant with GSD I is brought to medical attention as a result of tachypnea caused by lactic acidosis. Affected children are usually pale and pasty-looking with characteristic facies, often described as 'cherubic' owing to the doll-like appearance caused by the chubby cheeks. Truncal obesity and marked abdominal protuberance contrast with the typically thin extremities. Recurrent nosebleeds are common as a result of a secondary defect in platelet function; platelet numbers are usually normal.

In addition to hypoglycemia, laboratory examination typically shows lactic acidosis, hyperuricemia, hypertriglyceridemia, and hypophosphatemia. Serial measurements of plasma glucose show that the tolerance of fasting is poor, often less than three hours. The hypoglycemia is characteristically unresponsive to administration of glucagon. A distinguishing feature of GSD I is a significant rise in plasma lactate in response to glucagon. The kidneys are typically enlarged, and mild renal tubular dysfunction is common, though rarely clinically significant.

The basic defect in GSD I is deficiency of the production of glucose from glucose-6-phosphate, the final common pathway for glycogenolysis and gluconeogenesis (Figure 5.1). The commonest variant of the disease (type Ia) is caused by deficiency of the microsomal enzyme, glucose-6-phosphatase. The enzyme is only expressed in liver and kidney, and definitive diagnosis requires enzyme analysis of one or other tissue, usually liver. Liver biopsy shows massive glycogen accumulation, including glycogen within the nucleus of hepatocytes (Figure 5.4). In addition, there is marked accumulation of macrovesicular fat, but typically no fibrosis, evidence of biliary obstruction, or inflammation. Deficiency of glucose-6-phosphatase can often be demonstrated histochemically. However, the diagnosis should generally be confirmed by specific enzyme analysis on fresh liver obtained by biopsy.

The non-type Ia variants of GSD I are caused by deficiency in the microsomal transport of glucose-6-phosphate (type Ib), phosphate (type Ic), or glucose (type Id). Types Ib and Ic are clinically indistiguishable from type Ia. However, they are also associated with persistent neutropenia, and affected children typically have histories of recurrent pyogenic infections and pyorrhea.

Treatment of all types of GSD I is aimed primarily at preventing hypoglycemia by the administration of frequent low-fat feeds, containing as little fructose and galactose as possible. This is supplemented by intermittent ingestion of uncooked cornstarch during the day and tube feeding with formula during the night. The neutropenia in patients with non-type Ia disease responds well to treatment with granulocyte-colony stimulating factor (G-CSF).

The combination of hypoglycemia, marked hepatomegaly, and lactic acidosis is also characteristic of other defects of gluconeogenesis, such as hereditary fructose intolerance, fructose-1,6-diphosphatase deficiency, PEPCK deficiency, and sometimes in pyruvate carboxylase (PC) deficiency.

In patients with *hereditary fructose intolerance (HFI)*, the development of symptoms is clearly related to the ingestion of fructose or sucrose, often presenting with intractible vomiting, sometimes severe enough to suggest pyloric obstruction. Fructose ingestion often precipitates symptomatic hypoglycemia. More prolonged exposure results in failure to thrive, chronic irritability, hepatomegaly, abdominal distension, edema, and jaundice. Milder variants of the disease are common. Affected patients may complain of nothing more than sugar intolerance (bloating, abdominal discomfort, diarrhea).

In addition to hypoglycemia, marked lactic acidosis, hyperuricemia, and hypophosphatemia, affected patients have evidence of hepatocellular dysfunction (elevated aminotransferases, increased plasma methionine and tyrosine levels, prolonged prothrombin and partial thromboplastin times, hypoal-buminemia, hyperbilirubinemia), and renal tubular dysfunction (hyper-chloremic metabolic acidosis, generalized amino aciduria). The diagnosis is confirmed by demonstrating deficiency of aldolase B (fructose-1,6-bisphosphate aldolase) in fresh liver with fructose-1-phosphate and fructose-1,6-bisphosphate as substrates. Activities with both substrates are typically markedly decreased, although the effect with fructose-1-phosphate as substrate is more pronounced. Fructose tolerance tests in patients with HFI are *very dangerous* and should only be conducted under carefully controlled circumstances in patients who are in good general condition.

Fructose-1,6-diphosphatase deficiency may be difficult to differentiate from GSD Ia. In both diseases, the liver may be greatly enlarged. In fructose-1,6-diphosphatase deficiency, however, the reponse to glucagon is preserved. Definitive diagnosis requires measurement of the enzyme in fresh liver obtained by biopsy. Mitochondrial PEPCK deficiency is a very rare hereditary defect in gluconeogenesis associated with severe hypoglycemia, lactic acidosis, hepatomegaly, renal tubular dysfunction, hypotonia, and deteriorating liver function. Liver biopsy shows microvesicular steatosis and inflammatory changes. The diagnosis can be made by demonstrating deficiency of the enzyme in fibroblasts in which the mitochondrial isozyme predominates.

Over-utilization of glucose

The glucose utilization rate can be measured directly by the use of infusions of stable isotope-labeled glucose, but this is generally impractical except in centers actively involved in research on glucose metabolism. However, glucose oxidation rates can be estimated indirectly by determining the *minimum* rate of glucose administration needed to maintain euglycemia. This is relatively easy in neonates who are often receiving intravenous glucose. In older infants and children, the absence of ketones in the urine (determined by bedside Ketostix or Acetest tests on a few drops of urine), or depressed plasma 3-hydroxybutyrate levels, during hypoglycemia is usually a strong indication that glucose utilization is increased. Increased glucose utilization (i.e., hypoketotic hypoglycemia) occurs either as a result of hyperinsulinism, or as a result of a primary or secondary defect in fatty acid oxidation. The two situations are distinguishable by measurement of plasma free fatty acid levels. One of the most powerful physiologic effects of insulin is inhibition of hormone-sensitive lipase in adipose tissue. Low free fatty acid levels during hypoglycemia are a strong indication that insulin levels are abnormally elevated. By contrast, in patients with impaired fatty acid oxidation, free fatty acid levels are characteristically elevated. One way to quantitate this is to

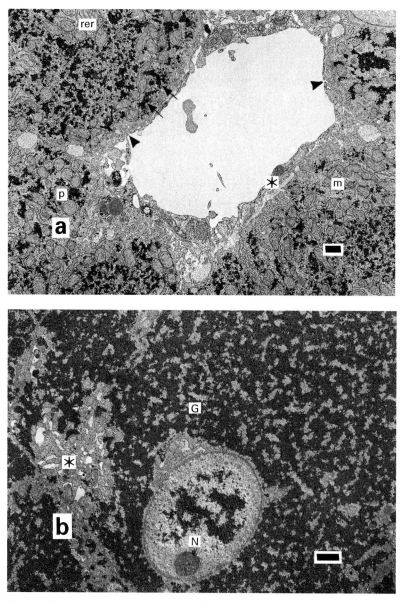

Fig. 5.4. Electron micrograph of normal liver (a) and liver in glycogen storage disease (b).

Figure **a**, shows normal liver. Portions of several normal hepatocytes surrounding a sinusoidal blood space are shown. The black deposits (arrows) in the cytoplasm of liver cells are glycogen aggregates. Mitochondira (m), peroxisomes (p) and rough

Table 5.2. *Approach to hypoketotic hypoglycemia.*

Tolerance of fasting (in hours)	Possible causes	Laboratory findings
Less than 1	Hyperinsulinism	Low plasma FFA levels with normal FFA/3-HOB ratio; high insulin/3-HOB ratio; high insulin/glucose ratio.
1–6	GSD type I; other defects in gluconeogensis	High plasma FFA levels with increased FFA/3-HOB ratio; lactic acidosis.
8–24	Fatty acid oxidation defects; systemic carnitine deficiency	High plasma FFA levels with very high FFA/3-HOB ratio; organic aciduria; low plasma carnitine levels.

Note: Abbreviations: FFA, free fatty acid; 3-HOB, 3-hydroxybutyrate; GSD, glycogen storage disease.

calculate the ratio of free fatty acids to 3-hydroxybutyrate (or to 3-hydroxybutyrate + acetoacetate). Hypoketotic hypoglycemia caused by hyperinsulinism is associated with a normal ratio (<2.0), while that associated with fatty acid oxidation defects is typically elevated (>3.0). In disorders of gluconeogenesis, including GSD I, the ratio is also often elevated as a result of secondary inhibition of ketogenesis. However, the timing of the hypoglycemia and other laboratory findings (Table 5.2) usually make differentiation of the conditions relatively straight forward.

In the face of a relative or absolute decrease in the capacity for mitochondrial fatty acid β-oxidation, fatty acids are oxidized by nonmitochondrial oxidative pathways to produce medium-chain (6- to 10-carbon length) dicarboxylic acids

Caption for Fig. 5.4 (*cont.*)

endoplasmic reticulum (rer) can also be seen. Note the endothelial cell processes (*) and fenestra (arrowheads). The bar represents 1 μm. Figure **b**, shows liver from a patient with glycogen storage disease, type Ia. Massive stores of electron dense glycogen particles (G) occupy the cytoplasm and displace mitochondria and other organelles (*) to the periphery of the cells. Glycogen can also be seen in the nucleus (N). The bar represents 1 μm. (Courtesy of Dr. M.J. Phillips.)

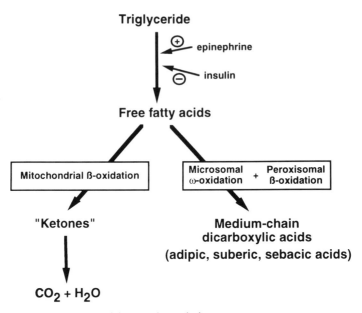

Fig. 5.5. Overview of fatty acid metabolism.

(Figure 5.5). This occurs when increased fatty acid oxidative flux exceeds the normal capacity for mitochondrial β-oxidation, or when normal mitochondrial fatty acid β-oxidation is impaired. The first is typically associated with marked ketonuria. In addition to hypoketotic hypoglycemia, patients with defects in mitochondrial fatty acid β-oxidation characteristically show medium-chain dicarboxylic aciduria, owing to increased nonmitochondrial fatty acid oxidation. However, in contrast to physiologic situations in which dicarboxylic aciduria is associated with severe ketosis, urinary 3-hydroxybutyrate and acetoacetate levels in patients with fatty acid oxidation defects are typically low. Putting it another way, a ratio of adipate to 3-hydroxybutyrate exceeding 0.5 is suggestive, though not diagnostic, of a mitochondrial fatty acid β-oxidation defect (see Chapter 4).

Inherited disturbances of fatty acid oxidation, such as systemic carnitine deficiency and MCAD deficiency, often present as acute and/or recurrent Reye-like syndrome: vomiting, lethargy, drowsiness, stupor, seizures, hepatomegaly, hypoglycemia, and hyperammonemia. These patients are particularly important to recognize because treatment is simple and effective and the natural history of the disorders in affected children surviving early childhood appears to be benign. Moreover, since the metabolic defects are hereditary, the siblings of affected children are at high risk for being similarly affected.

Table 5.3. *Relationship between metabolic defects and clinical manifestations of mitochondrial fatty acid β-oxidation defects.*

Pathophysiology	Clinical effects
Accumulation of intermediates of fatty acid oxidation (substrate accumulation)	Organic aciduria, acute encephalopathy, hepatocellular dysfunction, cardiac arrhythmias
Inability to meet the energy needs of tissues that are highly dependent on fatty acid oxidation for energy (deficiency of product)	Skeletal myopathy, cardiomyopathy
Requirement for tissues to draw on glucose oxidation to meet energy needs (secondary metabolic abnormalities)	Hypoglycemia
Secondary carnitine depletion (resulting from accumulation and excretion of acylcarnitines)	Hypoglycemia, hyperammonemia, myopathy, cardiomyopathy

Confirmation of the diagnosis of fatty acid oxidation defects can usually be obtained by demonstrating the presence of high concentrations of C-6 to C-10 dicarboxylic acids (adipic, suberic, and sebacic acids) in the urine during acute metabolic decompensation, the presence of characteristic acylcarnitines and/or acylglycines, and the presence of depressed free carnitine levels in plasma and/or urine. Since the organic acid abnormalities often disappear when the child is apparently healthy, diagnosis may be difficult if urine and blood samples are not saved from the time when the patient was acutely ill.

Hypoglycemia is a prominent secondary metabolic phenomenon in all mitochondrial fatty acid β-oxidation defects. However, each of the disorders is also associated with other problems arising from primary and secondary effects of the respective enzyme or transport deficiencies (Table 5.3). These are described in other chapters dealing with the most prominent clinical aspects of various defects, such as acute encephalopathy, chronic myopathy, or cardiomyopathy.

Hepatocellular dysfunction
Inherited metabolic diseases presenting as acute hepatocellular dysfunction present a particularly challenging diagnostic problem. The resemblance of some of them to acquired disorders, particularly viral infections and intoxications, is so close that discrimination on clinical grounds alone is next to impossible. Furthermore, hepatocellular dysfunction, regardless of the underlying cause, is

Table 5.4. *Inherited metabolic diseases presenting as severe hepatocellular dysfunction organized according to age of onset.*

Disease	Defect	Distinguishing features
Onset in the first few months of life		
Galactosemia	GALT	Severe hyperbilirubinemia; hemolytic anemia
Hepatorenal tyrosinemia	Fumarylacetoacetate hydrolase	Prominent coagulopathy; extreme elevation of AFP; succinylacetone in urine
LCHAD deficiency	LCHAD	'Hepatitis'; cardiomyopathy; dicarboxylic aciduria
α₁-Antitrypsin deficiency	α₁-Antitrypsin	Jaundice, failure to thrive; portal hypertension; GI hemorrhages
HFI	Aldolase B	Lactic acidosis; severe hypoglycemia
GSD, type IV	Glycogen brancher enzyme	Early, severe cirrhosis; myopathy
Wolman disease	Acid lipase	Severe failure to thrive; steatorrhea; calcification of adrenals
Peroxisomal disorders	Various disturbances of peroxisomal biogenesis or metabolism	Marked psychomotor retardation, hypotonia and weakness, seizures, cerebral dysgenesis and leukodystrophy
Mitochondrial depletion sydrome	mtDNA depletion	Severe hepatocellular dysfunction, myopathy, lactic acidosis
Onset later in infancy or early childhood		
GSD, type III	Glycogen debrancher enzyme	Skeletal myopathy
Gaucher disease, type III	Glucocerebrosidase	Massive hepatosplenomegaly; storage cells in marrow (see Fig 7.5).
Niemann-Pick disease, type C	Unknown	Neurodegenerative disease; storage cells in marrow; hepatosplenomegaly
CPT 1 deficiency	CPT 1	Hypoketotic hypoglycemia, elevated plasma carnitine levels
Onset in adolescence		
Wilson disease	Copper transporter ATPase	Acute 'hepatitis'; hemolysis; neuropsychiatric disturbances
CESD	Acid lipase	Hepatosplenomegaly; hypercholesterolemia
Adult onset		
Niemann-Pick disease, type B	Acid sphingomyelinase	Hepatosplenomegaly; storage cells in marrow; pulmonary infiltrates

Note: Abbreviations: HFI, hereditary fructose intolerance; CPT, carnitine palmitoyltransferase; CESD, cholesterol ester storage disease; GALT, galactose-1-phosphate uridyltransferase; GSD, glycogen storage disease; LCHAD, long-chain 3-hydroxyacyl-CoA dehydrogenase.

associated with secondary metabolic abnormalities that are often difficult to distinguish from the abnormalities observed in primary metabolic disorders. For example, increased concentrations of tyrosine in plasma are a common nonspecific metabolic manifestation of severe liver disease. Hypertyrosinemia is also typical of hepatorenal tyrosinemia. To make matters even more confusing, hepatorenal tyrosinemia commonly presents in early infancy as severe liver failure.

One way to approach this category of inborn errors of metabolism is to organize them according to age of onset. Inherited metabolic diseases characterized by severe liver disease may present in early infancy, later in childhood, or in adulthood (Table 5.4).

The presentation of inherited metabolic diseases with onset in the newborn period or early infancy as acute hepatocellular disease is characterized in most cases by some combination of failure to thrive, mild to severe hyperbilirubinemia, hypoglycemia, hyperammonemia, elevated transaminases, bleeding diathesis, edema, and ascites.

Persistent jaundice with marked conjugated hyperbilirubinemia, elevated aminotransferases, hepatosplenomegaly, and failure to thrive, dating from the first few weeks of life, is often the first indication of hepatic disease due to *α1-antitrypsin deficiency*. Cholestasis may be severe enough to cause acholic stools resembling those seen in infants with extrahepatic biliary atresia. Infants with liver disease due to α_1-antitrypsin deficiency develop cirrhosis with portal hypertension and may present at a few months of age with abdominal distension, ascites, marked hepatosplenomegaly, and upper gastrointestinal hemorrhage from esophageal varices. Despite the apparently aggressive nature of the disease, survival for many years with severe liver disease is not unusual. Liver biopsy shows typical PAS-positive, diastase-resistant inclusions within the endoplasmic reticulum of hepatocytes. Conventional electrophoresis of plasma proteins on cellulose acetate usually shows absence or marked deficiency of the alpha-1 protein peak. The diagnosis is confirmed by demonstrating the characteristic PI type ZZ phenotype on PI typing of plasma α_1-antitrypsin by isoelectric focusing or agarose gel electrophoresis of plasma proteins. Alternatively, the diagnosis can be confirmed by demonstrating homozygosity for the *PI*Z* allele by PCR amplification of genomic DNA from small samples of peripheral blood leukocytes.

Infants with *hepatorenal tyrosinemia* may present at a few weeks of age with acute hepatic failure progressing rapidly to death. More often, they present with a history of failure to thrive with intermittent episodes of marked anorexia, irritability, and drowsiness generally associated with intercurrent illnesses. As a

rule, they show only mild hyperbilirubinemia. The liver may not be particularly large, but it is usually hard and irregular to palpation, an indication of the extent of the fibrosis occurring early in the disease. Some ascites is common at presentation. Hypotonia and depressed deep tendon reflexes are an indication of peripheral neuropathy.

Affected infants usually show moderate to severe anemia and thrombocytopenia. Hypoglycemia is common, but plasma ammonium levels are usually not severely elevated. The transaminases may be only moderately elevated, but the coagulopathy is characteristically severe and typically associated with dysfibrinogenemia (reptilase time greater than the thrombin time). The renal tubular acidosis is more severe than that seen in infants with galactosemia. It is often associated with phosphate losses sufficient to cause rickets. Plasma amino acid analysis typically shows increased levels of tyrosine, methionine, and phenylalanine. However, the levels may not be much higher than those seen in patients with other types of severe hepatocellular disease; they are often not particularly helpful in making the diagnosis of tyrosinemia. But, the plasma α-fetoprotein (AFP) levels are characteristically extremely high. In fact, there are only a few situations in which comparable AFP levels are seen: hepatoblastoma, neonatal hemochromatosis, and resolving viral hepatitis are the main ones. Urinary organic acid analysis usually, though not always, shows the presence of succinylacetone, derived from fumarylacetoacetate accumulating proximal to the enzyme defect. If a diagnosis of hepatorenal tyrosinemia is stongly suspected, urinary organic acid analysis, including analysis of oxime derivatives (see Chapter 9), should be repeated at least three to four times. Definitive diagnosis is made by measuring fumarylacetoacetate hydrolase (FAH) activity in leukocytes, erythrocytes, fibroblasts, or liver tissue obtained by biopsy. Treatment with dietary tyrosine restriction often produces prompt clinical and metabolic improvement. However, plasma methionine levels often rise to levels exceeding 1 mmol/L during the early phases of treatment. The treatment of this condition has been revolutionized by the introduction of NTBC, an inhibitor of *p*-hydroxyphenylpyruvic acid dioxygenase (see Chapter 10).

Early-onset cirrhosis is also a prominent feature of *glycogen storage disease, type IV* (GSD IV). However, unlike α_1-antitrypsin deficiency, many patients also show evidence of neuromuscular involvement with hypotonia, weakness, muscle wasting, and depressed deep tendon reflexes. In fact, the disease in patients presenting later in life with milder variants of the condition is characterized by progressive skeletal myopathy, sometimes involving the myocardium (see Chapter 6). The course of typical early-onset disease is usually very aggressive, and survival beyond a few months is uncommon. Liver biopsy typically shows

advanced cirrhosis and the presence in hepatocytes of characteristic inclusions comprised of abnormal glycogen. The diagnosis is confirmed by measurement of glycogen brancher enzyme activity in leukocytes, fibroblasts, or tissue.

Some children with the subacute neuronopathic variant of *Gaucher disease (type III)* present in the first few years of life with massive hepatosplenomegaly and early evidence of chronic hepatic failure. In addition to hepatosplenomegaly, affected children show marked failure to thrive, protuberance of the abdomen, anemia, edema, ascites, and a bleeding diathesis out of proportion to the thrombocytopenia caused by hypersplenism. Death often occurs within a few years, before the underlying neuronopathic nature of the disease becomes obvious. Bone marrow aspirates show the presence of typical storage cells (see Chapter 7). The diagnosis is confirmed by demonstrating deficiency of β-glucosidase in leukocytes or fibroblasts.

Onset of clinically significant liver disease before age five years in patients with *Wilson disease* is unusual, though not unknown. Patients with this condition may present with hepatic syndrome, neurologic syndrome, or severe intravascular hemolysis. Some patients present with acute hepatitis, with jaundice, anorexia, general malaise, pale stools, and dark urine. The symptoms and routine laboratory findings are indistinguishable from those of acute viral hepatitis. Recovery is the rule, and the underlying defect often goes undetected at this stage. The absence of serologic evidence of viral infection, along with the presence of mild hemolytic anemia, should alert the clinician to the possibility of the disease.

Some patients, usually adolescents, present with an acute icteric hepatitis progressing over a period of several days to weeks to frank liver failure, with severe jaundice, hepatic coma, severe coagulopathy, ascites, renal failure, and death. The course of the illness and age of the patient often raises questions about severe viral hepatitis or intoxication. However, the presence of severe non-immune hemolytic anemia, caused by sudden release of copper from dying liver cells, is typical of this fulminant form of Wilson disease.

Presentation as 'chronic active hepatitis' may occur among adolescents and young adults with Wilson disease, with fatiguability, general malaise, anorexia, and hyperbilirubinemia, and tender enlargement of the liver. Sometimes the disease presents insidiously with signs of slowly progressive cirrhosis, including edema, gynecomastia, ascites, clubbing, or spider nevi. Some patients may have pathognomonic Kayser-Fleischer rings in the corneas. Laboratory studies show elevated aminotransferases and γ-globulin, decreased plasma albumin, and prolonged prothrombin time. Liver biopsy shows abnormalities typical of chronic active hepatitis, in addition to steatosis and periportal glycogenated

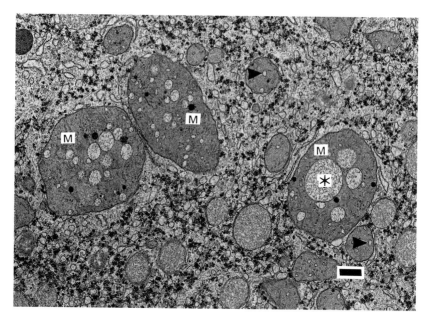

Fig. 5.6. Electron micrograph of liver in Wilson disease.
Greatly enlarged mitochondria (M) containing microcystic inclusion (*) and smaller dilated cristae in normal sized mitochondria (arrowheads) are shown. The latter is the most constant abnormality seen in liver of patients with Wilson disease. The bar represents 1 μm. (Courtesy of Dr. M.J. Phillips.)

nuclei, which are more suggestive of Wilson disease. Ultrastructural studies typically show mtiochondrial abnormalities characteristic of the disease (Figure 5.6).

Presentation of Wilson disease as a neuropsychiatric disorder is common, particularly among older adolescents and young adults. The clinical aspects of this presentation are discussed in Chapter 2. Most patients with neurologic Wilson disease also show some evidence of hepatic dysfunction.

Confirmation of the diagnosis may be difficult. In Wilson disease, plasma copper and ceruloplasmin levels are usually low. However, copper levels may be normal or elevated in patients with fulminant liver failure, and ceruloplasmin levels often overlap with those of patients with other types of liver disease. Urinary copper excretion is usually increased in Wilson disease, especially after administration of penicillamine. This is the basis of a diagnostic procedure widely used when the results of other studies are ambiguous.

Table 5.5. *Investigation of liver function.*

Tests of cholestasis	Investigation of inborn errors of metabolism
Bilirubin, conjugated and unconjugated	Copper and ceruloplasmin
Alkaline phosphatase (ALP)	α-Fetoprotein (AFP)
γ-Glutamyltranspeptidase (GGT)	α$_1$-Antitrypsin (PI phenotyping)
Bile acids	Plasma amino acids
	Urinary organic acids
Tests of active liver cell damage	Red cell GALT activity
Aspartate aminotransferase (AST)	Various lysosomal enzyme assays
Alanine aminotransferase (ALT)	
Tests of synthetic functions	
Albumin	
PT and PTT	
Coagulation factors VII, V	
Ammonium	

Note: Abbreviations: PT, prothrombin time; PTT, partial thromboplastin time; GALT, galactose-1-phosphate uridyltransferase.

Investigation

Liver function tests

Initial investigation might include a selection of studies to assess cholestasis, active liver cell damage, synthetic functions of the liver, and some selected studies that might be indicated by the nature of the hepatic presentation (Table 5.5).

Fasting tests

Carefully monitored fasting is one of the few provocative tests still widely used to screen for defects in carbohydrate or fat metabolism. It is undertaken to evaluate the integrity of glycogenolysis, gluconeogenesis, and fatty acid oxidation in the adaptation to starvation.

Any provocative testing should be conducted very carefully to avoid acute metabolic decompensation which might have disastrous results. Fasting as a provocative procedure should only be undertaken under controlled and closely monitored circumstances. Testing should be done when the patient is free of intercurrent illness.

In the investigation of severe hypoglycemia, or hypoglycemia occurring after only a few hours of fasting, such as is characteristic of GSD type I, the entire procedure can generally be completed in a few hours. After any feeding of the day, a secure intravenous is established with 0.9% NaCl infusing at a slow rate to maintain the line. The blood glucose is monitored periodically with the use of bedside test strips or glucometer until it drops to 2 mmol/l, until the child becomes symptomatic (usually with irritability, restlessness, sweating, or drowsiness), or until four to six hours have elapsed, depending on the age of the patient. At the termination of the fast, a sample of blood is obtained for measurement of blood glucose, lactate, free fatty acids, 3-hydroxybutyrate, acetoacetate, insulin, and growth hormone. Glucagon (1 mg) is then administered intramuscularly, and blood samples are obtained at 10, 20, and 30 minutes for analysis of glucose and lactate. In the event the child becomes severely symptomatic or refuses oral feedings at the end of the test, a bolus of glucose solution (500 mg/kg) should be administered intravenously and followed by a continuous glucose infusion.

In the absence of a clear history of hypoglycemia, or if the history indicates the child is able to tolerate at least several hours of fasting, fasting is begun from the evening feeding the day before: at 22.00 hours in children ≤ 18 months and at 18.00 hours in patients > 18 months of age. The blood glucose should be monitored periodically at the bedside during the night. At 08.00 hours, an intravenous of 0.9% NaCl is established and baseline analyses done of plasma glucose, lactate, free fatty acids, 3-hydroxybutyrate, ammonium, and free and total carnitine. After the patient has voided for the first time in the morning, all urine passed during the rest of the period of fasting is collected for urinary ketone and organic acid analysis. Blood glucose levels are monitored by bedside testing at hourly intervals. When the blood glucose falls to 2 mmol/L, the child becomes symptomatic, or after a total of 16 hours of fasting in children ≤ 18 months and 22 hours in children > 18 months of age, which ever comes first, blood is obtained for repeat analysis of plasma glucose, lactate, free fatty acids, 3-hydroxybutyrate, acetoacetate, and ammonium.

Provocative fasting as a test for defects in fatty acid oxidation has been abandoned by many centers because it is dangerous; some deaths have been attributed to metabolic decompensation occurring in the course of testing. Instead, many investigators rely on other methods to identify children requiring further investigation. Alternative testing procedures include carnitine or phenylpropionate loading coupled with analysis of acylcarnitines or phenylpropionate, respectively, in the urine. Loading in this situation is done only to ensure that the patient has adequate stores of carnitine, or is producing sufficient amounts of phenylpropionate in the gut, to produce the characteristic abnormalities in urine.

Bibliography

Bonnefont, J.P., Specola, N.B., Vassault, A., Lombes, A., Ogier, H., de Klerk, J.B.C., Munnich, A., Coude, M., Paturneau-Jouas, M. & Saudubray, J.-M. (1990). The fasting test in paediatrics: application to the diagnosis of pathological hypo- and hyperketotic states. *European Journal of Pediatrics*, **150**, 80-5.

CPC of the Massachusetts General Hospital (MGH 44-1984). (1984). A 15-year-old girl with possible chronic active hepatitis. *New England Journal of Medicine*, **311**, 1170–7.

Dunger, D.B. & Leonard, J.V. (1982). Value of the glucagon test in screening for hepatic glycogen storage disease. *Archives of Diseases of Childhood*, **57**, 384–9.

Guzmán, M. & Geelen, M.J.H. (1993). Regulation of fatty acid oxidation in mammaliam liver. *Biochimica et Biophysica Acta*, **1167**, 227–41.

Kelly, D. & Green, A. (1991). Investigation of pediatric liver disease. *Journal of Inherited Metabolic Diseases*, **14**, 531–7.

Lake, B.D. (1991). The role of histochemical investigation in metabolic disorders affecting the liver. *Journal of Inherited Metabolic Diseases*, **14**, 538–45.

Phillip, M., Bashan, N., Smith, C.P.A. & Moses, S.W. (1987). An algorithmic approach to diagnosis of hypoglycemia. *Journal of Pediatrics*, **110**, 387–90.

Pollitt, R.J. (1995). Disorders of mitochondrial long-chain fatty acid oxidation. *Journal of Inherited Metabolic Diseases*, **18**, 473–90.

Pons, R. & De Vivo, D.C. (1995). Primary and secondary carnitine deficiency syndromes. *Journal of Child Neurology*, **10** (Suppl. 2), 2S8–24.

Rebouche, C.J. & Engel, A.G. (1983). Carnitine metabolism and deficiency. *Mayo Clinic Proceedings*, **58**, 533–40.

Stanley, C.A. (1987). New genetic defects in mitochondrial fatty acid oxidation and carnitine deficiency. *Advances in Pediatrics*, **34**, 59–88.

Suchy, F.J. (ed.) (1994). *Liver Disease in Children*. St. Louis: Mosby-Year Book, Inc.

Talente, G.M., Coleman, R.A., Alter, C., Baker, L., Brown, B.I., Cannon, R.A., *et al.* (1994). Glycogen storage disease in adults. *Annals of Internal Medicine*, **120**, 218–26.

Tsalikian, E. & Haymond, M. (1983). Hypoglycemia in infants and children. In: *Hypoglycemic Disorders*, ed. F.J. Service, pp. 35–71. Boston: GK Hall Medical Publishers.

6

Cardiac syndromes

Until recently, the contribution of inherited metabolic diseases to conditions presenting primarily with symptoms of cardiac disease would have been considered to be small, and devoting an entire chapter of a clinical text like this to them would have been considered unusual. However, over the past 10 years, presentation as serious cardiac disease has become associated in particular with two types of inherited metabolic disorders, inborn errors of fatty acid oxidation and mitochondrial electron transport chain (ETC) defects. Clinically significant cardiac involvement is also now recognized to be a serious complication, if not the presenting problem, in patients with some inherited metabolic diseases in which it was previously unknown, rare, or trivial.

Cardiomyopathy

Many of the inherited metabolic disorders in which cardiac disease is particularly prominent present as cardiomyopathy (Table 6.1). The clinical characteristics of the cardiomyopathy itself are often not much help in determining whether it is the result of an inborn error of metabolism or some nonmetabolic condition, such as infection or intoxication. Moreover, even among the inherited metabolic diseases, the clinical characteristics of the cardiac involvement are usually not characteristic enough to suggest a specific diagnosis without further investigation.

In most inherited metabolic diseases presenting with cardiomyopathy, echocardiography shows some thickening of the left ventricular wall. However, in some, notably in patients with systemic carnitine deficiency, the marked enlargement of the heart seen on radiographs of the chest is principally the result of dilatation. Cardiac enlargement and dilatation is commonly accompanied by arrhythmias and by valvular abnormalities, such as mitral insufficiency and mitral valve prolapse, regardless of the underlying cause.

From the standpoint of making a specific clinical diagnosis of inherited metabolic cardiomyopathy, regardless of the underlying defect, the most important features of the various conditions in which it occurs are the associated noncardiac findings. The myocardium is muscle, and most inherited metabolic conditions affecting the metabolism of cardiocytes also affect skeletal muscle, at least to some extent. The presence of clinically significant *myopathy* is, therefore, an important clue to the metabolic nature of the underlying defect. In some cases, such as glycogen storage disease, type II (GSD II or Pompe disease), the skeletal myopathy is profound; in others, like long-chain 3-hydroxyacyl-CoA dehydrogenase (LCHAD) deficiency, it may be relatively subtle and difficult to differentiate from nonspecific weakness and hypotonia owing to the severity of the heart disease. Skeletal muscle biopsy is often helpful, if not diagnostic, in many of these disorders, particularly the mitochondrial myopathies (see Chapter 2).

The presence of hepatomegaly may be a clue to a systemic defect in glycogen or fatty acid metabolism (see Chapter 5), bearing in mind that enlargement of the liver, often with some evidence of hepatocellular dysfunction, is a prominent nonspecific sign of heart failure in young infants. Marked hepatomegaly without evidence of severe hepatocellular dysfunction is characteristic of all the hepatic glycogen storage diseases, except GSD IV (brancher enzyme deficiency) in which cirrhosis generally occurs early and clinically significant cardiomyopathy is relatively rare. It is of some interest, particularly in the light of the discovery of patients with late-onset disease apparently limited to the heart, that children with GSD IV without apparent heart involvement may develop fatal dilated cardiomyopathy some years after the hepatic glycogen storage disease is cured by liver transplantation. Cardiomyopathy is a relatively common, though rarely clinically significant, problem in patients with GSD III (debrancher enzyme deficiency).

The presence of severe hepatocellular dysfunction is a classic characteristic of fatty acid oxidation defects, including many patients with systemic carnitine deficiency (see Chapter 5). In fact, patients with systemic carnitine deficiency, long-chain acyl-CoA dehydrogenase (LCAD) or LCHAD deficiency are about equally split between those presenting as a hepatic syndrome and those presenting as cardiomyopathy. Interestingly, cardiomyopathy does not occur in patients with medium-chain acyl-CoA dehydrogenase (MCAD) deficiency. As a rule, among patients with other fatty acid oxdiation defects, the older the patient, the more likely they are to present with cardiomyopathy. However, even in these, evidence of hepatocellular dysfunction is generally obvious. This includes enlargement of the liver, elevated transaminases, and decreased plasma carnitine levels with increased ratio of esterified to free carnitine. In LCAD deficiency and LCHAD deficiency, urinary organic acid analyses done when the patient is

Table 6.1. *Inherited metabolic diseases in which cardiomyopathy is prominent.*

Disease	Other clinical features
Disorders of glycogen metabolism and glycolysis	
Pompe disease (GSD II)*	Profound skeletal myopathy presenting in early infancy; early death
GSD III (debrancher enzyme deficiency)	Hepatomegaly, variable hypoglycemia, mild hepatocellular dysfunction
GSD IV (brancher enzyme deficiency)*	Hepatic involvement may initially be mild in variants with major cardiac involvement
Phosphorylase *b* kinase deficiency*	Cardiomyopathy may be the only problem
Triosephosphate isomerase deficiency	Chronic hemolytic anemia, progressive dystonia, spasticity; early death
Disorders of fatty acid metabolism	
Systemic carnitine deficiency*	Skeletal myopathy, Reye-like episodes of acute encephalopathy
LCAD deficiency*	Skeletal myopathy, exercise intolerance with myoglobinuria, Reye-like episodes of acute encephalopathy
LCHAD deficiency*	Intermittent acute hepatocellular dysfunction
Carnitine-acylcarnitine translocase	Early-onset acute encephalopathy, hypotonia, hyperammonemia, seizures, hepatomegaly and hepatocellular dysfunction, heart block
Organic acidopathies	
Propionic acidemia*	Intermittent acute metabolic acidosis, ketosis, hyperammonemia, neutropenia
Methylmalonic acidemia	Intermittent acute metabolic acidosis, ketosis, hyperammonemia, neutropenia
HMG-CoA lyase deficiency	Intermittent acute metabolic acidosis, hypoglycemia, hyperammonemia, neutropenia
Mitochondrial acetoacetyl-CoA thiolase (β-ketothiolase) deficiency	Intermittent severe metabolic acidosis, ketosis, hypoglycemia, hyperammonemia
Glutaric acidemia type II (multiple acyl-CoA dehydrogenase deficiency)	Facial dysmorphism, congenital malformations, hypotonia, hepatomegaly, hypoketotic hypoglycemia, metabolic acidosis, hyperammonemia
Amino acidopathies	
Hepatorenal tyrosinemia	Acute hepatocellular dysfunction, hypoglycemia, renal tubular acidosis, porphyria
Alkaptonuria†	Dark urine, calcification of cartilage, arthritis
Homocystinuria†	Marfanoid habitus, psychomotor retardation, dislocation of lens, thromboembolic phenomena
Mitochondrial cardiomyopathies	
Kearns-Sayre syndrome*	External ophthalmoplegia, retinal degeneration, cerebellar ataxia, growth failure, sensorineural deafness, heart block

Disease	Features
Lethal infantile cardiomyopathy*	Cardiac dysrhythmias (e.g., WPW syndrome); early death
Leigh disease (subacute necrotizing encephalomyelopathy)	Psychomotor retardation, hypotonia, failure to thrive, breathing abnormalities, oculomotor disturbances, seizures, lactic acidosis
Hypertrophic cardiomyopathy and myopathy*	Skeletal myopathy, diabetes mellitus, cataracts, cardiac dysrhythmia (e.g., WPW syndrome)
Barth syndrome*	Skeletal myopathy, chronic neutropenia, 3-methylglutaconic aciduria
Benign infantile mitochondrial myopathy and cardiomyopathy	Weakness, hypotonia, respiratory failure, severe lactic acidosis, cardiomyopathy, variable course
MELAS	Psychomotor retardation, growth failure, seizures, stroke-like episodes, lactic acidosis
MERRF	Cerebellar ataxia, skeletal myopathy, psychomotor retardation, myoclonus, seizures

Glycosphingolipidoses, mucopolysaccharidoses, and glycoproteinoses

Disease	Features
Fabry disease*	Chronic and recurrent neuritic pain in hands and feet, peculiar skin lesions, corneal opacities, progressive renal failure, cardiac dysrhythmias, premature cerebrovascular disease; X-linked recessive
Hurler disease (MPS IH)*	Facial dysmorphism, hepatosplenomegaly, dysostosis multiplex, progressive psychomotor retardation, corneal clouding, MPSuria
Hunter disease (MPS II)	Facial dysmorphism, hepatosplenomegaly, dysostosis multiplex, progressive psychomotor retardation, MPSuria; X-linked recessive
Maroteaux-Lamy disease (MPS VI)	Short stature, dysostosis multiplex, corneal clouding, normal intelligence, MPSuria
GM1 gangliosidosis*	Facial dysmorphism, hepatosplenomegaly, ± dysostosis multiplex, oligosacchariduria
GM2 gangliosidosis	Chronic progressive encephalopathy, seizures, cherry-red spots in retinal, blindness
Gaucher disease	Hepatosplenomegaly, anemia, thrombocytopenia, bone crises
Niemann-Pick disease	Hepatosplenomegaly, chronic progressive encephalopathy
I-cell disease	Hurler-like appearance, hepatosplenomegaly, dysostosis multiplex
Juvenile neuronal ceroid-lipofuscinosis	Psychomotor regression, seizures, progressive visual impairment

Note: Abbreviations: MPS, mucopolysaccharidosis; MPSuria, mucopolysacchariduria; GSD, glycogen storage disease; LCAD, long-chain acyl-CoA dehydrogenase; LCHAD, long-chain hydroxyacyl-CoA dehydrogenase; HMG-CoA, 3-hydroxy-3-methylglutaconyl-CoA; WPW, Wolff-Parkinson-White; MELAS, mitochondrial encephalomyopathy, lactic acidosis, and stroke-like episodes; MERRF, myoclonic epilepsy and ragged red-fiber disease.

* Cardiomyopathy may be dominant or only clinical problem.
† Cardiomyopathy probably the result of chronic ischemic heart disease.

acutely ill show the presence of medium- and long-chain dicarboxylic acids and, in LCHAD deficiency, long-chain (C12 and C14) 3-hydroxy monocarboxylic and dicarboxylic acids (see Chapter 4). The organic acid abnormalities are characteristically evanescent and may not be present by the time urine is collected for analysis. Confirmation of the diagnosis requires the demonstration of the relevant fatty acid oxidation defect in fibroblasts. Hepatocellular dysfunction, skeletal myopathy, metabolic acidosis, and dysmorphism are also generally more prominent than the myocardial involvement in patients with cardiomyopathy resulting from multiple acyl-CoA dehydrogenase deficiency (glutaric acidemia type II; GA II). However, occasionally, cardiomyopathy develops as an early and fatal complication.

Hepatosplenomegaly is a prominent and diagnostically important associated finding in patients with cardiomyopathies occurring as a result of mucopolysaccharide or other storage conditions. Patients with Hurler disease (MPS IH) may present at three to five months of age in frank congestive heart failure as a result of infiltration of the myocardium with glycosaminoglycan. Although the liver and spleen are characteristically palpably enlarged, these signs, along with the characteristic coarse facial appearance and dysostosis multiplex, are subtle at this age, and they may be missed. Severe cardiomyopathy in the other neurovisceral storage diseases, like Niemann-Pick disease, is rare, and the presence of the associated neurologic and somatic abnormalites is usually obvious. What is important to bear in mind here is that sudden deterioration of a patient with one of these conditions may be the result of cardiomyopathy.

Neurologic abnormalities (including skeletal myopathy) are characteristic of the multisystem involvement that is typical of the mitochondrial myopathies in which cardiomyopathy may dominate the presentation (see Chapter 2). The cardiomyopathy in patients with mitochondrial ETC defects is almost always hypertrophic, and it is often associated with conduction abnormalities and arrhythmias (reviewed later). In some instances, the noncardiac manifestations of a mitochondrial cytopathy may be insignificant. Because the disorder often affects members of every generation, shows transmission from parents to children, and affects both sexes equally, the cardiomyopathy may be concluded to be the result of an autosomal dominant genetic defect. However, a carefully recorded family history in these cases will show that the disorder is transmitted as a matrilineal trait, from mothers to offspring, but not through fathers, characteristics typical of mitochondrial cytopathies.

Table 6.2. *Initial investigation of a possible inherited metabolic cardiomyopathy.*

Histology unknown (i.e., before endocardial biopsy)
Depending on the results of clinical examination, ECG, chest radiograph, and echocardiography:

Blood
   Blood gases and plasma electrolytes (calculate anion gap; see Chapter 4)
   Plasma lactate
   Plasma amino acid analysis
   Plasma carnitine, free and total
   Plasma acylcarnitines
   Plasma ammonium
   Leukocyte α-glucosidase, β-galactosidase, and β-hexosaminidase

Urine
   Urinary organic acids
   Urine carnitine and acylcarnitines
   Urinary MPS and oligosaccharide screens

Other
   Closely monitored, prolonged fast with measurements of urinary organic acids, plasma free fatty acids, 3-hydroxybutyrate, lactate, pyruvate, and glucose (see Chapter 5)

Histological evidence of 'lipid myopathy' or 'mitochondrial disorder'
In addition to the above:
Skeletal muscle biopsy for histology, histochemistry, and electron microscopy, as well as biochemical studies, such as measurement of muscle carnitine and evaluation of mitochondrial electron transfer
Skin biopsy for enzymic studies on cultured fibroblasts
Liver biopsy for histology, electron microscopy, and enzyme analyses

Note: Abbreviations: MPS, mucopolysaccharide.

Initial investigation of possible inherited metabolic cardiomyopathy

Because of the clinical overlap in the cardiac manifestations of various inherited metabolic diseases, the initial diagnostic laboratory workup of a patient presenting with a cardiomyopathy should include the examination of several possibilities (Table 6.2).

Endocardial biopsy is often helpful in the differential diagnosis of cardiomyopathy, including that occurring as a result of inborn errors of metabolism. In addition to the routine assessment of inflammatory changes and a search for viral particles, specimens should be examined by electron microscopy for evidence of submicroscopic mitochondrial lesions. Specific microscopic changes may be very subtle and obscured by the presence of secondary pathological changes, such as endocardial fibroelastosis. Three types of microscopic change are particularly helpful in suggesting the presence of an inborn error of metabolism, but they are not always present:

- Evidence of intralysosomal storage of macromolecules is characteristic of lysosomal storage diseases, and the histochemical and ultrastructural characteristics of the stored material provides guidance for further, more specific, diagnostic investigation. In conditions like GSD II, Fabry disease, and late-onset neuronal ceroid-lipofuscinosis, the histochemical and electron microscopic changes are generally sufficiently typical to suggest the specific diagnosis. In others, like Niemann-Pick disease, the changes are either nonspecific or too dispersed to be reliably identifiable in the small samples of tissue obtainable by this technique.

- The presence of significant amounts of microvesicular neutral lipid, demonstrable by Oil Red O or Sudan Black B staining of frozen sections, or by electron microscopy, is characteristic of disorders of fatty acid oxidation, such as systemic carnitine deficiency, LCHAD deficiency, and Barth syndrome. The changes in the myocardium of patients with fatty acid oxidation defects may be very subtle. One of our patients with confirmed LCHAD deficiency showed only modest inflammatory change in an endocardial biopsy; there was no evidence of neutral lipid accumulation.

- The presence of markedly increased numbers of mitochondria, which are characteristically aggregated immediately under the sarcolemma and are often enlarged and structurally abnormal, is characteristic of the cardiomyopathy associated with mitochondrial ETC defects. In some cases, mitochondrial proliferation is so great that it causes enlargement of muscle fibers, producing the appearance of histiocyte-like cells, sometimes called oncocytic or 'histiocytoid' cardiomyopathy. Abnormal intracellular accumulation of glycogen and neutral fat is also a feature of mitochondrial cardiomyopathies. In other cases, some increase in the number of mitochondria and the accumulation of some glycogen and neutral fat occur as nonspecific changes with chronic hypoxemia. Marked accumulation of cytosolic glycogen in cardiocytes may be the only clue to the nature of the underlying disease in infants with a particularly virulent variant of phosphorylase b kinase deficiency, apparently limited to the heart, presenting in the newborn period with dilated or hypertrophic cardiomyopathy and progressing rapidly to death. Some patients with variants of GSD IV (brancher enzyme deficiency) also present with cardiac glycogenosis with only subtle hepatic involvement.

Systemic carnitine deficiency

Patients with systemic carnitine deficiency coming to attention in the first few months of life often present with hypoketotic hypoglycemia, hyperammonemia, and other evidence of hepatocelluar dysfunction (see Chapter 4); the cardiomyopathy is not the predominant problem, though it is usually present. In contrast, cardiomyopathy is often the primary problem in children presenting after a year of age with the disease. The cardiomyopathy is usually progressive, and it is associated with weakness and hypotonia resulting from skeletal muscle involvement. Measurement of plasma carnitine levels is usually diagnostic. Although carnitine levels may be nonspecifically depressed in patients with cardiomyopathy, regardless of the underlying cause, in patients with primary systemic carnitine deficiency, plasma levels are generally extremely low (<10 μmol/L). Moreover, the response to treatment with large doses of oral L-carnitine is usually dramatic, with significant improvement in myocardial function occurring within a few days. Severe secondary carnitine depletion is a characteristic feature of many inborn errors of organic acid metabolism (see Chapter 4), some of which may present as cardiomyopathy. Therefore, the investigation of any infant or child presenting in this manner should also include analysis of urinary organic acids. In children with primary systemic carnitine deficiency, the urinary organic acid profile is generally normal.

Glycogen storage disease, type II (GSD II or Pompe disease)

The massive hypertrophic cardiomyopathy of *Pompe disease (GSD II)* is rarely confused with other causes of cardiomyopathy in infants. The ECG shows huge QRS complexes, marked left-axis deviation, shortening of the PR interval, and T-wave inversion. The liver is often palpably enlarged as a result of congestive heart failure, not hepatic glycogen storage. Skeletal muscle involvement is generally obvious (see Chapter 2). The diagnosis is confirmed by demonstrating profound deficiency of α-glucosidase (acid maltase) in leukocytes or fibroblasts. Urinary oligosaccharide analysis often shows abnormalities, but these are not sufficiently specific to establish the diagnosis. Although the cardiac disease is severe, death is usually the result of respiratory failure because of the skeletal myopathy.

Fabry disease

Cardiac involvement in patients with Fabry disease is usually associated with diagnostically important noncardiac signs, such as the peculiar skin lesions, severe neuritic pain in the hands and feet, and progressive renal disease, which dominate the clinical presentation of the disease. However, in some, the cardiac findings are the only clinically significant manifestations of the disease. Left ventricular hypertrophy and mitral insufficiency, as a result of accumulation of globotriaosylceramide (GL-3) in the myocardium and mitral valve, are consistent features in adolescents and young adult males with this X-linked disorder of glycolipid metabolism. Conduction abnormalities (progressive shortening of the PR interval) and arrhythmias (intermittent supraventricular tachycardia) are also common, though rarely clinically significant.

Arrhythmias

Arrhythmias are a common, relatively nonspecific complication of the cardiomyopathy in patients with inherited metabolic diseases regardless of the underlying metabolic disorder. Varying degrees of heart block or other conduction defects and associated dysrhythmias, such as Wolff-Parkinson-White preexcitation syndrome, occur in a variety of otherwise unrelated inherited metabolic cardiomyopathies, such as Kearns-Sayre syndrome (a mitochondrial cytopathy), Fabry disease (a lysosomal storage disease), carnitine-acylcarnitine translocase (a fatty acid oxidation defect), and propionic acidemia (an organic acidopathy), to list only a few. However, in some conditions, disturbances of cardiac rhythm are particularly prominent, even fatal. Heart block is particularly common in patients with Kearns-Sayre syndrome, and it may develop before the characteristic noncardiac features of the disease are recognized.

Coronary artery disease
Familial hypercholesterolemia
Premature coronary artery disease is the hallmark of familial hypercholesterolemia (FH). The condition is caused by defects in the uptake and metabolism of circulating cholesterol, the most common being mutations affecting the amount or the properties of the cell surface receptor for plasma low density lipoprotein (LDL). The lipids in plasma are transported in association with specific apoproteins (Table 6.3). LDL uptake is mediated by LDL receptor-mediated endocytosis and fusion of the endosome with lysosomes where the cholesterol is de-esterified and the apoprotein is broken down to its constituent amino acids. The unesterified cholesterol exits the lysosome and enters the cytosol where it is used for the synthesis of membranes. It also down-regulates the local production of LDL receptor and the activity of 3-hydroxy-3-methyl-glutaryl-CoA (HMG-CoA) reductase, the most important enzyme in the regulation of cholesterol biosynthesis. LDL receptor defects cause impaired

uptake of the lipoprotein resulting in enhanced intracellular biosynthesis of the lipid as well as retention of the cholesterol-rich lipoprotein in the circulation. The result is marked increases in the concentration of LDL-cholesterol in plasma and early development of atherosclerosis.

FH is one of the most common mendelian genetic diseases, affecting about one of every 500 individuals in Western countries like the U.S. It is transmitted as an autosomal dominant condition. Heterozygotes generally present in their late twenties or thirties with coronary artery disease, often fatal myocardial infarction. Homozygotes have severe hypercholesterolemia and often present in early childhood, or even as infants, with ischemic heart disease, including myocardial infarction, and evidence of cholesterol accumulation in other tissues, particularly the skin. Myocardial infarction in infants is manifested by tachypnea, sweating, pallor, and the appearance of apprehension. In older children, cholesterol in the skin and other tissues produces typical tuberous xanthomas on the extensor surfaces of the extremities (Figure 6.1), arcus senilis, xanthelasma, subcutaneous nodules, and thickening of the Achilles tendons. Patients with this condition usually have a strong family history of premature ischemic heart disease. Measurement of fasting plasma lipids typically reveals total cholesterol levels in excess of 6.5 mmol/L in heterozygotes and 15 mmol/L in homozygotes. The excess cholesterol is accountable by increased levels of LDL; VLDL (very low density lipoprotein) levels are generally only modestly elevated, and high density lipoprotein (HDL) levels are often decreased.

Abnormalities of plasma lipids are features of a number of primary disorders of lipoprotein metabolism, many of which are associated with an increased risk of premature coronary artery disease (Table 6.4). The investigation of hyperlipidemia requires careful attention to the circumstances of testing and consideration of the large number of conditions in which secondary hyperlipidemia occurs. In general, secondary hyperlipidemia is much more common than primary disorders of plasma lipoprotein metabolism. Plasma lipid analyses should be done on blood obtained after an over-night fast and after at least three days abstention from alcohol. Lipid analyses should include measurement of total triglycerides, total cholesterol, LDL-cholesterol, and HDL-cholesterol (see Chapter 9). Note should be made of any medications, dietary fat intake, obesity, and history of medical conditions, such as diabetes, kidney disease, and hypothyroidism. Testing should routinely include tests of thyroid and kidney function.

Tuberous xanthomatosis is seen in patients with *sitosterolemia*, a disorder of plant sterol metabolism, which is characterized by premature coronary atherosclerosis, intermittent hemolysis or chronic hemolytic anemia, and recurrent arthritis of the knees and ankles. In patients with sitosterolemia, the plasma apo

Table 6.3. *Plasma lipoproteins.*

Lipoprotein	Apoproteins	Protein (% of dry wt)	Lipids (% of dry wt)			Function
			TG	PL	C + CE	
Chylomicrons	**Apo B-48, C-I, C-II** Apo A-I, A-IV, C-III, E	1	90	5	4	Transport of absorbed triglyceride from gut. Triglyceride is hydrolyzed by endothelium-bound LPL in adipose tissue and muscle; Apo A and Apo C transferred to HDL. Chylomicron remnants taken up by liver.
VLDL	**Apo B-100, C-I, C-II & C-III** Apo A-I, A-II, E	8	55	19	20	Transport of triglyceride synthesized in liver to adipose tissue and muscle; Apo C transferred to HDL. About half the VLDL is converted into LDL in liver.
LDL	**Apo B-100** Apo C-I, C-II, C-III, E	20	5	20	55	Transport of cholesterol from the liver to peripheral tissues.
HDL	**Apo A-I, A-II** Apo C-I, C-II, C-III, E	50	5	27	21	Transport of cholesterol from peripheral tissues to liver.

Note: Abbreviations: VLDL, very low-density lipoproteins; LDL, low-density lipoproteins; HDL, high-density lipoproteins; TG, triglyceride; PL, phospholipid; C + CE, sum of cholesterol and cholesterol ester. Bold type indicates principal apoprotein species.
Source: Data are from Bachorik & Kwiterovich (1991).

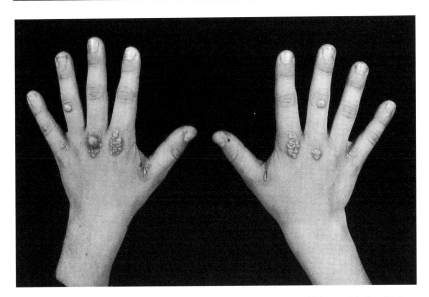

Fig. 6.1. Tuberous xanthomas on the hands of a seven-year-old boy with familial hypercholesterolemia.

B-100 concentrations may be elevated, but the plasma cholesterol is either normal or only moderately increased. Tendinous xanthomatosis is one of the primary clues to the diagnosis of *cerebrotendinous xanthomatosis*, a disorder characterized clinically by onset in adolescence of progressive neurologic deterioration (see Chapter 2).

Premature coronary artery disease is a major feature of Fabry disease in which accumulation of globotriaosylceramide (GL-3) in the walls of small arteries and arterioles predisposes to coronary atherosclerosis, myocardial ischemia, and myocardial infarction. Stroke may also occur as a result of cerebrovascular involvement. The same deposition in vessels of the skin and mucous membranes causes the pathognomonic skin lesions of the disease, angiokeratoma corporis diffusum.

Table 6.4. *Familial hyperlipidemias.*

Lipid abnormality	Type	Primary defect	Associated clinical features	Secondary disorders
Exogenous hyperlipidemia (↑↑Chylomicrons)	I	Familial LPL deficiency Apo C-II deficiency	Eruptive xanthomatosis, lipemia retinalis, acute pancreatitis, dyspnea, recent memory loss	Dysglobulinemias SLE
Endogenous hyperlipidemia (↑VLDL)	IV	(a) Familial hypertriglyceridemia (b) FCH (c) Tangier disease	(a) Eruptive xanthomatosis, lipemia retinalis, acute pancreatitis, dyspnea, recent memory loss (b) Premature coronary artery disease (c) Enlarged orange tonsils, splenomegaly, peripheral neuropathy	Many conditions, including: GSD type I Uremia Nephrotic syndrome Diabetes mellitus* Alcoholism* Estrogens* Glucocorticoids* Stress*
Mixed hyperlipidemia (↑VLDL + chylomicrons)	V	Familial hypertriglyceridemia Familial LPL deficiency	Eruptive xanthomatosis, lipemia retinalis, acute pancreatitis, dyspnea, recent memory loss	The same conditions as cause secondary type IV hyperlipidemia
Hypercholesterolemia (↑↑LDL)	IIa	FH FCH	Premature coronary artery disease, tuberous xanthoma, tendinous xanthomas, arcus senilis	Nephrotic syndrome Hypothyroidism Dysglobulinemias Cushing syndrome AIP

Combined hyperlipidemia ($\uparrow$LDL + VLDL)	IIb	FCH	Premature coronary artery disease	Nephrotic syndrome Hypothyroidism Dysglobulinemias Cushing syndrome Glucocorticoids* Stress*
Remnant hyperlipidemia (β-VLDL)	III	Familial dysbetalipoproteinemia	Tuberous and tuberoeruptive xanthomas, planar xanthomas, premature coronary artery disease, peripheral vascular disease	Hypothyroidism SLE

Note: Abbreviations: VLDL, very low-density lipoproteins; LDL, low-density lipoproteins; SLE, systemic lupus erythematosus; FCH, familial combined hyperlipidemia; AIP, acute intermittent porphyria; LPL, lipoprotein lipase; FH, familial hypercholesterolemia; GSD, glycogen storage disease.

* Conditions which by themselves do not cause hyperlipidemia, but often aggravate a primary hyperlipidemia.

Source: Data taken from Havel & Kane (1995).

Bibliography

Bachorik, P. & Kwiterovich, Jr., P.O. (1991). Measurement of plasma cholesterol, low-density lipoprotein cholesterol, and high-density lipoprotein cholesterol. In *Techniques in Diagnostic Human Biochemical Genetics: A Laboratory Manual*, ed. F.A. Hommes, pp. 425–59. New York: Wiley-Liss, Inc.

Böhles, H., Hofstetter, R. & Sewell, A.C. (Eds.) (1995). *Metabolic Cardiomyopathy*. Stuttgart: Wissenschaftliche Verlagsgesellschaft mbH.

Gilbert-Barness, E. (1989). Metabolic cardiomyopathy of childhood. In *Topics in Pediatrics: a festschrift for Lewis A. Barness*, ed. H.H. Pomerance & B.B. Bercu, pp. 122–53. New York: Springer-Verlag.

Guenthard, J., Wyler, F., Fowler, B. & Baumgartner, R. (1995). Cardiomyopathy in respiratory chain disorders. *Archives of Disease in Childhood*, **72**, 223–6.

Havel, R.J. & Kane, J.P. (1995). Introduction: structure and metabolism of plasma lipoproteins. In *The Metabolic and Molecular Bases of Inherited Disease*, 7th edn., ed. C.R. Scriver, A.L. Beaudet, W.S. Sly & D. Valle, pp. 1841–51. New York: McGraw-Hill, Inc.

Kelly, D.P. & Strauss, A.W. (1994). Inherited cardiomyopathies. *New England Journal of Medicine*, **330**, 913–19.

Kohlschutter, A. & Hausdorf, G. (1986). Primary (genetic) cardiomyopathies in infancy. A survey of possible disorders and guides for diagnosis. *European Journal of Pediatrics*, **145**, 454–9.

Marin-Garcia, J. & Goldenthal, M.J. (1994). Cardiomyopathy and abnormal mitochondrial function. *Cardiovascular Research*, **28**, 456–63.

Servidei, S., Bertini, E. & DiMauro, S. (1994). Hereditary metabolic cardiomyopathies. *Advances in Pediatrics*, **41**, 1–32.

7

Storage syndrome and dysmorphism

Over the years, the distinction between what was conventionally regarded as dysmorphic syndromes and inborn errors of metabolism has become blurred by the recognition that the consequences of many inborn errors of metabolism include physical features, such as facial dysmorphism, which would almost certainly be regarded as developmental defects if the nature of the underlying metabolic defect were not known. In fact, the recent discovery of a specific metabolic defect in patients with Smith-Lemli-Opitz (SLO) syndrome, a classical dysmorphic syndrome, has led to the suggestion that perhaps all hereditary dysmorphic syndromes should be regarded similarly – as inborn errors of metabolism – in which, however, the specific metabolic defect has not yet been identified. At the other extreme, if the physical features of Hurler disease, resulting directly from abnormal accumulation of the substrate of a defective enzyme, are regarded as 'dysmorphic', then perhaps any inherited metabolic disease showing physical abnormalities as a result of substrate accumulation should be regarded as a dysmorphic syndrome. The issue is raised to underscore the fact that the distinction between the two types of disorders is breaking down, and various biochemical and metabolic studies are being employed increasingly by clinical geneticists in the investigation of dysmorphism, particularly in infants presenting acutely ill early in life. The questions to be addressed in this chapter are:

- Are there characteristics of the dysmorphism which should prompt metabolic investigation?
- What are the types of inherited metabolic diseases in which dysmorphism might be expected to be prominent?
- What sort of metabolic studies are most likely to be diagnostically productive in the investigation of dysmorphism?

General characteristics of the dysmorphism resulting from inborn errors of metabolism

Developmental physical abnormalities in general have been classified as congenital malformations (primary dysmorphogenesis; poor formation), deformations (structural abnormalities resulting from mechanical interference with growth), and disruptions (structural abnormalities resulting from destructive processes). The mechanism of the dysmorphism occurring as a result of inborn errors of metabolism varies from one disorder to another. A few, like SLO syndrome, clearly involve disturbances of morphogenesis (malformation). In most, the distortion arises primarily as a result of a combination of deformation and disruption. The mucopolysaccharide storage diseases are good examples. Mucopolysaccharide accumulation causes abnormalities of shape, growth, and the physical properties, of any tissue normally containing significant amounts of connective tissue ground substance, such as bone, cartilage, ligaments, skin, blood vessels, dura mater, and heart valves (deformation). However, abnormalities of shape and growth also occur as a result of secondary destructive processes (disruption).

With this in mind, some generalizations can be made concerning the characteristics of the dysmorphism in many inherited metabolic diseases:

- The dysmorphic features associated with inborn errors of metabolism are generally disturbances of shape, rather than fusion or cellular migration abnormalities, or abnormalities of number (such as polydactyly).
- The dysmorphism tends to become more pronounced with age.
- Microscopic and ultrastructural abnormalities are often prominent.

There are some important exceptions. For example, cellular migration abnormalities are a prominent feature of the cerebral dysmorphogenesis occurring in many infants with Zellweger syndrome, glutaric aciduria type II, and pyruvate dehydrogenase (PDH) deficiency. Fusion abnormalities and abnormalities of number (e.g., polydactyly) are major, though not constant, features of SLO syndrome.

In many inherited metabolic disorders, the facies may be recognized to be unusual, though in a relatively nonspecific or very subtle way. Infants with PDH deficiency, for example, are mildly dysmorphic, though not in a way that is sufficiently characteristic to suggest the diagnosis. Generally, the peculiarities of the face are matters of proportion, rather than major structural abnormalities. Unrelated patients with the same disorder often look enough alike to appear to be related, but are not regarded as unusual or dysmorphic by themselves. For example, infants with Tay-Sachs disease generally have very attractive, fine,

Table 7.1. *Classification of inborn errors with significant dysmorphism.*

Lysosomal disorders	Peroxisomal disorders
Mucopolysaccharidoses	Zellweger syndrome and variants
MPS I (Hurler & Scheie diseases)	Rhizomelic chondrodysplasia punctata
MPS II (Hunter disease)	Adult Refsum disease
MPS III (Sanfilippo disease)	*Mitochondrial disorders*
MPS IV (Morquio disease)	PDH deficiency
MPS VI (Maroteaux-Lamy disease)	Glutaric aciduria, type II
MPS VII (Sly disease)	3-Hydroxyisobutyric aciduria
Glycoproteinoses	Mitochondrial ETC defects
Infantile sialidosis	*Biosynthetic defects*
Galactosialidosis	Mevalonic aciduria
Fucosidosis	SLO syndrome
α-Mannosidosis	CDG syndrome
β-Mannosidosis	Albinism
Aspartylglucosaminuria	Primary defects in hormone biosynthesis
Sphingolipidoses	Primary disorders of collagen biosynthesis
GM1 gangliosidosis	Homocystinuria*
Farber lipogranulomatosis	Menkes disease*
Combined defects	Alkaptonuria*
I-cell disease	*Receptor defects*
Multiple sulfatase deficiency	Familial hypercholesterolemia
	Pseudohypoparathyroidism
	Other hormone receptor defects

Note: Abbreviations: MPS, mucopolysaccharidosis; PDH, pyruvate dehydrogenase; ETC, electron transport chain; CDG, carbohydrate-deficient glycoprotein; SLO, Smith-Lemli-Opitz.
* The biosynthetic defect in these conditions is secondary to the metabolic consequences of the primary inborn error of metabolism.

doll-like, facial features. The same has been noted about patients with glycogen storage disease, type I, who are often described as resembling 'cupie dolls' owing to their chubby cheeks. Children with multiple sulfatase deficiency tend to have fine, attractive, facial features. With a few exceptions, the peculiarities of the face in these conditions are not sufficiently striking or specific to be diagnostically helpful. However, the physician may be alerted to the possibility by determining that the child does not resemble any other member of the family very closely, something that is often elicited by asking who the child takes after in the family, or by examining photos of their parents or siblings taken at about the same age.

What are the types of inherited metabolic diseases in which dysmorphism might be expected to be prominent?

Most of the inherited metabolic diseases associated with dysmorphism involve defects in organelle metabolism, biosynthetic processes, or receptor defects (Table 7.1). In some cases, serious structural defects, such as major neuronal migration abnormalities, are present at birth. Except for defects of hormone biosynthesis, which represent a special case, the response of all of them to treatment by environmental manipulation, including enzyme replacement in the few in which it has been attempted, is incomplete at best, even when the accumulating substrate of the defective reaction is water-soluble and diffusible (e.g., PDH deficiency).

What follows are brief descriptions of some of the more common inherited metabolic diseases in which dysmorphism is a major feature. They are organized according to the organelle or process involved.

Lysosomal disorders

Except for the uncommon instances in which lysosomal disorders present in the newborn period with non-immune fetal hydrops (see Chapter 8), the dysmorphic features in patients with inborn errors of lysosomal enzyme activity are usually not clinically obvious at birth, even though ultrastructural changes in tissues may be present as early as 20 weeks of gestation. Many of these disorders are characterized by the development, during infancy and early childhood, of 'storage syndrome'.

Storage syndrome

Storage syndrome is a constellation of clinical findings suggesting accumulation of macromolecular material in various tissues causing distortion of shape and growth manifested as:

- characteristic facies;
- bone changes (dysostosis multiplex) and short stature;
- organomegaly (megalencephaly, hepatosplenomegaly).

Although affected infants are usually considered normal at birth, a history of large birth weight associated with peripheral edema, sometimes severe enough to cause non-immune fetal hydrops, may be elicited. The onset of symptoms and awareness that something is wrong is usually gradual. Recurrent bouts of otitis media and persistent mucous nasal discharge are common, but rarely are they sufficiently different from what a normal child might experience to generate suspicion of the presence of a storage disorder before the development of other signs of disease.

Affected children may come to attention in a number of ways. The otolaryngologist, consulted because of the recurrent otitis media or persistent nasal discharge, may be the first to notice that the child has unusual facial features suggestive of a genetic disorder. Others come to attention because of abnormalities of growth, either excessively rapid growth of the head, suggesting the possibility of hydrocephalus, or growth retardation causing short stature. The incidental detection of hepatomegaly or hepatosplenomegaly often prompts further investigation. Sometimes the child comes to attention as a result of the investigation of developmental delay or extraordinarily difficult behavior. Occasionally the characteristic skeletal abnormalities are found incidentally on plain radiographs obtained because of suspected lower respiratory tract infections.

The face in patients with storage syndrome shows subtle changes which become more pronounced with age, but at such a slow rate, that parents often do not notice them. The changes include relative macrocephaly with prominence of the forehead, prominence of the brow, some puffiness of the eyelids, broadening and flattening of the bridge of the nose, anteverted nares, and thick upper lip. The general impression is one of 'coarse' facial features (Figures 7.1a–h). The hair is usually particularly coarse, and the pinnae of the ears are generally fleshy. The tongue is enlarged with some exaggeration of the fissuring. The teeth, which generally erupt on schedule, are often small, widely spaced, and dysplastic. The gums may be thickened. Clouding of the cornea is a feature of many of the inherited metabolic diseases presenting as storage syndrome, though it is generally only clinically obvious in the mucopolysaccharidoses, Hurler disease, Scheie disease, and Maroteaux-Lamy disease.

A prominent feature of virtually all the inherited metabolic diseases presenting with storage syndrome is short stature. Linear growth may actually be accelerated during the first year of life. However, growth during the second year slows suddenly, often arresting completely or showing little further gains after three to five years of age. The axial skeleton is shortened and often shows lumbar kyphosis. In Hurler disease (MPS IH), the kyphosis, caused by wedging of lumbar vertebrae, is often acute, producing the characteristic 'gibbus' deformity of the spine. Careful examination often shows limitation of active and passive movement of various joints, particularly the shoulders, elbows, fingers, and hips. Restriction of elevation of the arm at the gleno-humeral joint often occurs early. Limitation of active and passive movement of the elbows is also early and includes restriction of extension of the joint, as well as supination

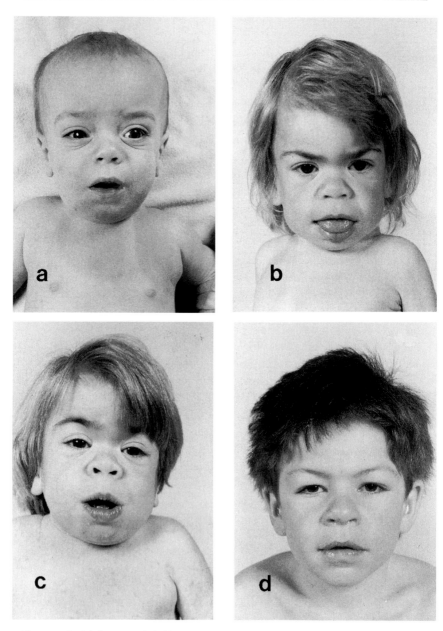

Fig. 7.1. Facial features of children with various lysosomal storage disorders. Panels **a**, Hurler disease (MPS IH) at four months of age; **b**, MPS IH at three years of age; **c**, MPS IH at seven years of age; **d** Hunter disease (MPS IIHA) at seven

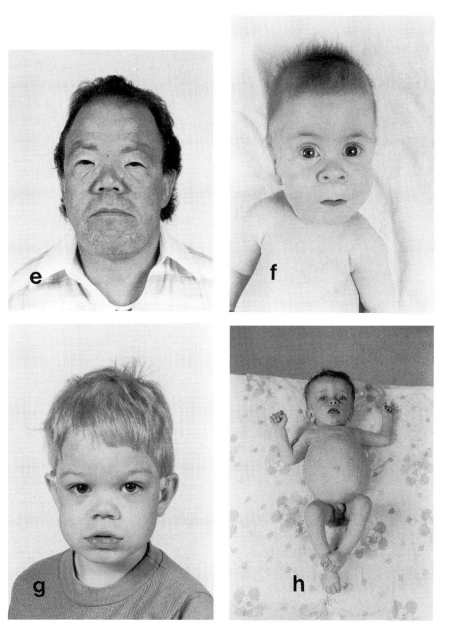

years of age; **e** Hunter disease (MPS IIB) at 42 years of age; **f**, seven-month-old infant with I-cell disease; **g** Mannosidosis at 5 years of age; **h**, 11-month-old boy with Niemann-Pick disease, type A.

and pronation. Limitation of extension of the hips results in a characteristic crouched standing posture with flexion at the knees and exaggerated lordosis of the lumbar spine. The fingers generally appear thickened and short, and they gradually become fixed in a partially flexed position over a period of several months or years. Similar changes occur in the toes, producing hammer-toe deformities.

Morquio disease (MPS IV) is a prominent exception to the generalized and severe restriction of joint movement seen in patients with most mucopolysac- charide storage diseases. In this condition, abnormalities of the skeleton dominate the clinical picture; hepatosplenomegaly is usually mild or absent, and mental retardation is rare. More than any of the other inherited metabolic diseases presenting with storage syndrome, Morquio disease closely resembles a nonmetabolic spondylo-epiphyseal dysplasia. In marked contrast to all the other MPS disorders, the joints in Morquio disease show abnormally *increased* mobility. The instability caused by hypermobility of joints interferes with efficient muscle action producing an impression of muscle weakness severe enough to suggest a primary myopathy.

Plain radiographs show widespread changes typical of mucopolysaccharide storage diseases in general, but not generally specific for any one in particular (Figures 7.2a–d). The skull is enlarged and thickened, and the sella turcica is enlarged (Figure 7.2a). Lateral radiographs of the thoraco-lumbar spine show flattening of the vertebrae, beaking of the antero-inferior lip, and often posterior displacement of one or more upper lumbar vertebrae (Figure 7.2b). Radiographs of the hands show shortening and broadening of the metacarpals and phalanges, producing a rounded, bullet-like shape, with generalized under-mineralization and increased coarse trabeculation (Figure 7.2d). The ilia of the pelvis are externally rotated and the acetabula are poorly formed (Figure 7.2c). Radio- graphs of the upper cervical spine in patients with Morquio disease, type A or type B, show hypoplasia or absence of the odontoid process producing instability of the atlanto-axial joint which can be appreciated by comparing lateral radiographs of the neck in flexion and extension.

In many of the lysosomal disorders presenting as storage syndrome, examin- ation of a routine, Wright-stained peripheral blood smear shows the presence of metachromatic granulation of mononuclear cells called Alder-Reilly bodies (Figure 7.3). However, this sign must be differentiated from the nonspecific granulation occurring in various acquired conditions, such as viral infections, and it is often absent, particularly in the the relatively mild MPS variants. Examination of bone marrow aspirates often shows the presence of storage histiocytes even if they are not present in the peripheral blood.

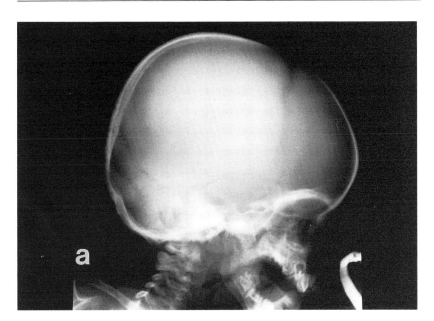

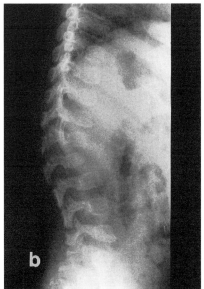

Fig. 7.2. Radiographs of patient with Hurler disease (MPS IH).
Figure **a**, lateral radiograph of the skull of a one-year-old child showing thickened calvarium and enlarged sella; Figure **b**, lateral radiograph of the thoraco-lumbar spine of a 14-month-old child showing flattening, beaking, and posterior

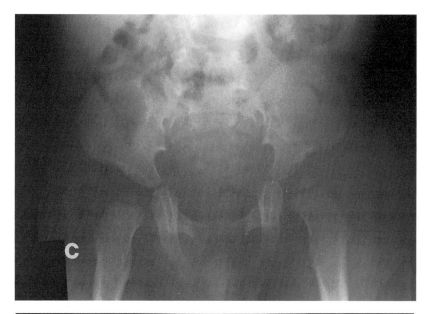

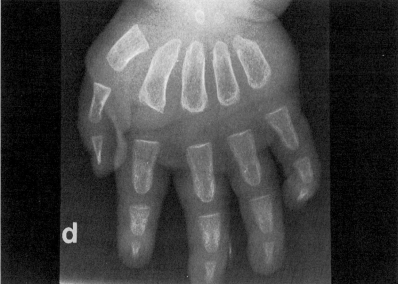

Figure 7.2 (*cont.*). displacement of vertebrae; Figure **c**, radiograph of the pelvis of a 14-month-old child showing flaring of the ilia of the pelvis and poor formation of the acetabula bilaterally; Figure **d**, radiograph of the hand of a 14-month-old child showing coarse thickening of the phalanges and metacarpals which have a typical bullet-shaped appearance.

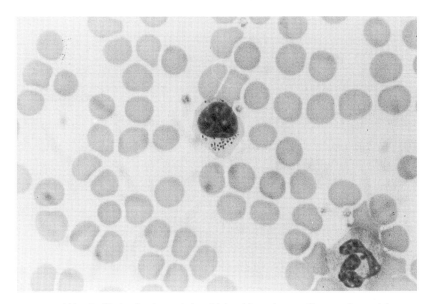

Fig. 7.3. Alder-Reilly bodies in peripheral blood lymphocyte from patient with Hurler disease (MPS IH). (Courtesy of Dr. Annette Poon.)

Some of the major clinical features of different lysosomal disorders presenting as storage syndrome are summarized in Table 7.2.

A number of conditions are commonly confused with inherited lysosomal disorders presenting as storage syndrome. Infants with congenital virus infections, such as congenital CMV or rubella, often present with a history of developmental delay, failure to thrive, and hepatosplenomegaly. The presence of generalized lymphadenopathy or chorioretinitis are features which help to differentiate this group of conditions from inborn errors of metabolism presenting as storage syndrome. Appropriate serological and virus isolation studies are generally sufficient to confirm the diagnosis of congenital infection. Disseminated neuroblastoma in young infants is often associated with hepatosplenomegaly. Unusual involuntary eye movements (i.e., opsiclonus) might suggest a metabolic neurodegenerative condition. The true nature of the underlying disease is usually revealed by examination of bone marrow smears showing the presence of neoplastic, not storage, cells. Histiocytosis X is another malignant condition which clinically may initially be confused with a storage disorder. Hepatosplenomegaly, along with pallor, developmental delay, and blindness, is characteristic of osteopetrosis. The skeletal radiographs in osteopetrosis are so characteristic that confusion with one of the lysosomal storage

Table 7.2. Some clinical features of lysosomal disorders presenting as 'storage syndrome'.

Disorder	Facies	Neurologic	Dysostosis multiplex	Eye findings	Hepatosplenomegaly	Other
Mucopolysaccharidoses						
MPS IH (Hurler)	Coarse	Severe MR	+++	Corneal clouding	+++	Death by age 10 years
MPS IH/S (Hurler-Scheie)	Coarse	± MR	Corneal clouding	+	Intermediate between MPS IH and MPS IS	
MPS IS (Scheie)	'Normal'	0	++	Corneal clouding	+	Short stature
MPS II (severe) (Hunter)	Coarse	Severe MR	+++	0	++	Death in late teens, often cardiac
MPS II (mild) (Hunter)	Coarse	0	++	0	+	Short stature
MPS III (Sanfilippo)	Mild coarsening	Severe MR	±	Corneal opacities	0	Severe behaviour abnormalities
MPS IV (Morquio)	Unusual	0	+++	Corneal opacities	0	Hypoplasia/absence of odontoid process
MPS VI (Maroteaux-Lamy)	Mild coarsening	± MR	++	Corneal clouding	±	Short stature
MPS VII (Sly)	Mild coarsening	Severe MR	++	?	+	Highly variable phenotype
Glycoproteinoses						
Infantile sialidosis	Coarse	MR	+++	CRS	±	Renal tubular acidosis

Juvenile sialidosis				CRS		
Galactosialidosis		MR, myoclonus	+ -+++	CRS	0	Angiokeratoma
Fucosidosis, type I (severe)	Mild coarsening	MR, seizures	++	–	++	Increased sweat chlorides
Fucosidosis, type II (mild)	Mild coarsening	MR	++	Telangiectasia	+	Angiokeratoma
α-Mannosidosis, type I	Coarse	Severe MR	+++	Cataracts, corneal opacities	+++	Early sensorineural hearing loss
α-Mannosidosis, type II	Mild coarsening	MR	++	Cataracts, corneal opacities	++	Early sensorineural hearing loss
Aspartylglucosaminuria	Mild coarsening	MR	+	Mild cataracts	0	Photosensitivity, acne
Sphingolipidoses						
GM1 gangliosidosis (infantile)	Coarse	Severe MR	++	± CRS	++	Early visual failure; hyperacusis
GM1 gangliosidosis (juvenile)	Normal	Moderate MR	±	0	0	Spasticity, ataxia

Note: Abbreviations: MR, mental retardation; CRS, cherry-red spot; +, present; ±, variably present; 0, absent.

diseases is impossible. Massive hepatosplenomegaly and failure to thrive are characteristics of familial erythrophagocytotic lymphohistiocytosis (FEL) which often suggest storage disease. However, the bone marrow findings are generally typical, showing histiocytosis and marked erythrophagocytosis.

Gaucher disease, type I

Non-neuronopathic Gaucher disease should be considered high on the list of diagnostic possibilities in any patient of any age presenting with asymptomatic splenomegaly or hepatosplenomegaly. It is particularly common among Ashkenazi Jews in whom the prevalence may be as high as 1 in 1000. Gaucher disease is a lysosomal storage disease caused by deficiency of acid glucocerebrosidase, called β-glucosidase when activity is measured using a synthetic substrate. It is characterized by intracellular accumulation of glucocerebroside in macrophages throughout the reticuloendothelial system, especially in the spleen, liver, bone marrow, and lungs. The symptoms of disease are directly related to the tissue distribution of the pathology.

The commonest presentation of the disease is asymptomatic splenomegaly or complications of hypersplenism. Unusual bruising, excessive bleeding during dental surgery, or postpartum hemorrhage may be the first indication of marked thrombocytopenia. Affected individuals usually have a sallow complexion and mild to moderate normocytic, normochromic anemia and mild neutropenia, and they often complain of fatiguability. Discovery of the anemia often prompts treatment with iron, even though bone marrow studies generally show ample, or even excessive, iron stores. The splenomegaly may become massive. Spleen weights in excess of 2 kg are not unusual. Enlargement of the spleen and liver often cause protuberance of the abdomen. Occasionally, patients experience bouts of excruciating abdominal pain related to the development of splenic infarcts.

Infiltration of the bone marrow with glucocerebroside-containing storage cells causes expansion of the marrow compartment producing thinning of the cortex and a characteristic widening of the ends of long bones. This produces a typical Erlenmeyer flask shape in the distal end of the femurs (Figure 7.4). Spontaneous fractures are common as a result of thinning of the cortex of bone throughout the body. One of the most debilitating complications of the disease are 'bone crises' characterized clinically by the sudden onset of very severe, localized pain, swelling, tenderness, heat, and redness, usually in one of the long bones of the lower extremities, usually associated with fever. Clinically, the appearance may be indistinguishable from osteomyelitis or septic arthritis, though cultures are generally negative. The crises generally resolve over a period of a few days. Radiologically, there may be nothing to see apart from soft-tissue swelling until

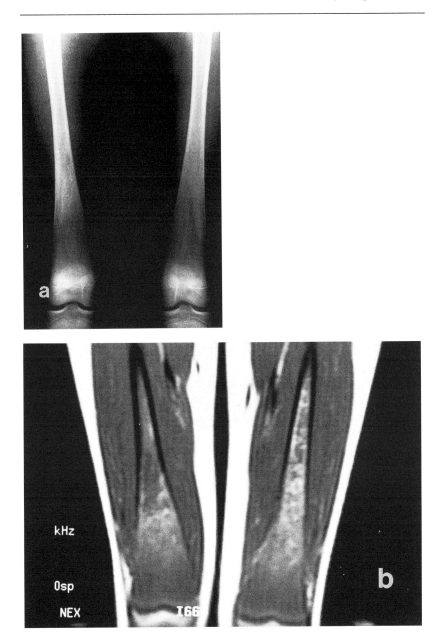

Fig. 7.4. Radiograph of the lower extremities in Gaucher disease.
Figure **a**, a plain radiograph showing typical thinning of cortex and expansion of the marrow cavity producing a characteristic Erlenmeyer flask appearance of the distal femurs. Figure **b**, an MRI scan showing mottled signal from the distal femurs (TR450/TE16). (Courtesy of Dr. Paul Babyn.)

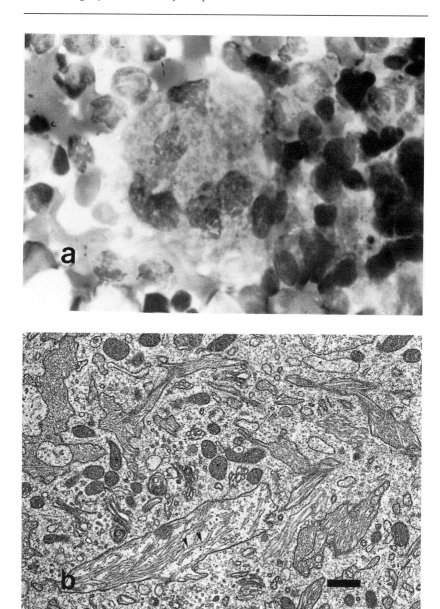

Fig. 7.5. Typical storage macrophage in the bone marrow of a patient with Gaucher disease.

Figure **a**, a photomicrograph showing the characteristic crinkled tissue paper appearance of Gaucher storage cells. (Courtesy of Dr. Annette Poon.) Figure **b**, an well after the pain has resolved. Sclerosis of bone in the area then follows. The pathophysiology of these episodes is unknown, though the clinical features suggest a vascular mechanism. Avascular necrosis of the heads of the femurs and humeri is also a common and debilitating complication of the disease. Clinical lung involvement is uncommon.

Bone marrow aspirates generally show the presence of typical Gaucher storage cells (Figure 7.5). The diagnosis is confirmed by demonstrating deficiency of β-glucosidase in peripheral blood leukocytes or cultured fibroblasts. Occasionally, similar storage cells are seen in the marrow of patients with Hodgkins disease or other lymphomas. The diagnosis is made even more challenging because peripheral blood leukocytes of patients with these lymphomas often have markedly depressed β-glucosidase activity. However, the activity in fibroblasts in patients with tumors is normal, and the β-glucosidase activity in peripheral blood leukoctyes characteristically returns to normal levels when the tumor regresses with treatment. Mutation analysis is becoming increasingly applied to the diagnosis of Gaucher disease, particularly among Jews, because a high proportion of the disease is associated with a relatively small number of mutant alleles.

Farber lipogranulomatosis

Classical *Farber lipogranulomatosis*, an autosomal recessive sphingolipid storage disorder caused by deficiency of the lysosomal enzyme, ceramidase, is characterized by onset in the first few weeks to months of life of painful swelling of joints, particularly of the distal extremities, subcutaneous nodules, a hoarse cry and respiratory distress, failure to thrive, and fever. Lymphadenopathy and moderate hepatomegaly may also occur, but splenomegaly is rare. One of our patients had massive hepatomegaly, evidence of significant hepatocellular dysfunction, and ascites. Affected infants are typically irritable and appear apprehensive, particularly during handling, which causes pain. Most, though not all, show psychomotor retardation; some have seizures. Generalized muscle weakness, atrophy, and hypotonia are associated with decreased or absent deep tendon reflexes. Eye abnormalities are common; an atypical cherry-red spot is seen in many. The course of the disease is relentlessly progressive, with increasing inanition owing to feeding difficulties, the development of joint contractures,

Caption for Fig 7.5 (*cont.*)

electron photomicrograph showing part of a Kupffer cell. The tubule-like structures (arrowheads) shown within the lysosomes of this cell are diagnostic of Gaucher disease. The bar represents 0.5 μm. (Courtesy of Dr. M.J. Phillips.)

increasing pulmonary infiltration and respiratory difficulties, and death, usually within a few months.

Milder variants of the disease are less common than the classical disease and are characterized by long-term survival, many with apparently normal intelligence. Some patients present in the newborn period with very aggressive disease in which hepatosplenomegaly is prominent and death occurs within a few weeks to months. Massive histiocytic infiltration of lungs, liver, spleen, and thymus, along with the common absence of subcutaneous nodules in infants with this malignant variant of the disease, may be misdiagnosed as malignant histiocytosis. Rarely, patients with Farber lipogranulomatosis present at one to three years of age with psychomotor regression and rapidly progressive neurodegeneration, prominent macular cherry-red spots, ataxia, quadriparesis, seizures, and death within several months to a few years. The presence of subcutaneous nodules is an important clue to the clinical diagnosis.

Histopathologic studies on tissues affected in Farber disease show accumulation of histiocytes with secondary fibrosis. Some of the lesions progress to form well-organized granulomas with macrophages, lymphocytes, and multinucleated giant cells surrounding a central core of foamy, PAS-positive, storage histiocytes. The diagnosis is confirmed by demonstrating acid ceramidase deficiency in tissues, including peripheral blood leukocytes, or cultured fibroblasts. This is one lysosomal hydrolase which must be measured using the natural substrate of the enzyme; synthetic, fluorogenic substrates do not work. This limits the immediate availability of the test to laboratories providing specialized biochemical diagnostic services.

Peroxisomal disorders
Zellweger syndrome

Infants with classical *Zellweger syndrome*, caused by a defect in peroxisome biogenesis, display physical characteristics which are so specifically characteristic of the condition that diagnosis is usually possible on inspection alone. The face is typical. It is characterized by a high and prominent forehead, hypoplastic supraorbital ridges, epicanthic folds, and depressed and broad root of the nose (Figure 7.6). Affected infants show typically profound hypotonia and weakness, severe feeding difficulties, very large fontanelles and wide cranial sutures, redundant skin folds of the neck, abnormal external ears, eye abnormalities (nystagmus, corneal clouding, Brushfield spots, glaucoma, cataracts, or pigmentary retinopathy), seizures, single palmar creases, and hepatomegaly.

Abdominal ultrasound examination almost always shows cystic disease of the kidneys, and often increased echogenicity of the liver. Plain radiographs often

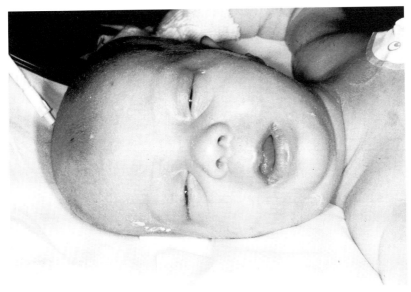

Fig. 7.6. Facial features of a newborn infant with classical Zellweger syndrome.

show calcific stippling of the patella and synchondrosis of the acetabulum (Figure 7.7). CT and MRI studies of the brain typically show disorganization of the cerebral cortex and white matter abnormalities indicative of severe myelin deficiency (Figure 7.8).

Electron microscopic examination of liver obtained by biopsy shows absence of peroxisomes. Biochemical studies reveal multiple abnormalities of peroxisomal function (see Chapter 9). Measurement of plasma very long-chain fatty acids is generally the most accessible and reliable biochemical test for confirming the diagnosis.

Numerous nonclassical variants of Zellweger syndrome have been encountered, each showing some of the characteristics of the classical disease. On the basis of clinical differences between them, some have been separated off as different diseases, such as *neonatal adrenoleukodystrophy* (NALD) and *infantile Refsum disease* (IRD). However, as the number of patients recognized as having peroxisomal defects has increased, the distinction between clinically similar syndromes has become blurred. Moreover, on the basis of complementation studies many patients with different clinical phenotypes would appear to be genetically indistinguishable. Zellweger syndrome, NALD, and IRD may all represent different positions on a clinical continuum associated with different

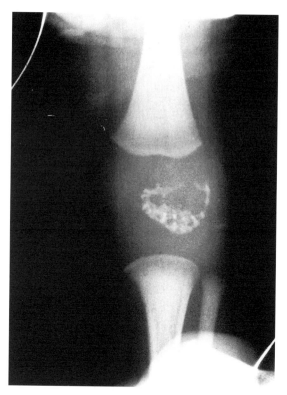

Fig. 7.7. Radiograph of the knee in a patient with Zellweger syndrome showing stippling of the patella.

mutations in the same gene. The results of the same type of complementation studies also indicate that marked genetic heterogeneity exists *within* distinct clinical phenotypes, such as classical Zellweger syndrome. Many of the disorders have certain characteristics in common which should alert the clinician to the possibility of a peroxisomal disorder. These are features which are prominent in Zellweger syndrome, and collectively they are here called the *severe peroxisomal phenotype*. They include:

- marked psychomotor retardation;
- profound hypotonia and weakness;
- intractible seizures;
- sudanophilic leukodystrophy;
- hepatocellular dysfunction;

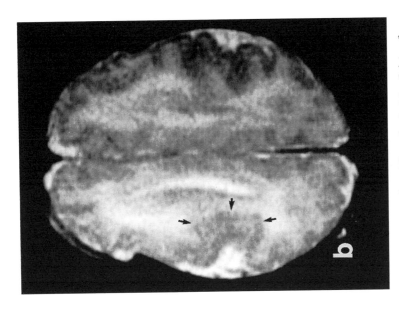

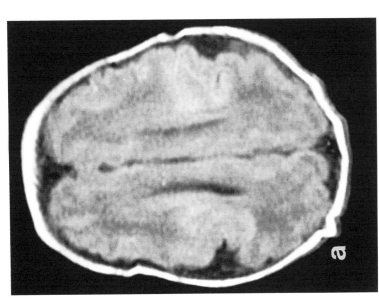

Fig. 7.8. MRI scan of the brain in patient with Zellweger syndrome. MRI scans of the brain show bilateral primitive Sylvian fissures lined by thickened, grossly abnormal cerebral cortex (arrows, Figure **b**), and poorly formed gyrae throughout. Figure **a**, T1-weighted scan (TR600/TE20); Figure **b**, T2-weighted scan (TR3000/TE120). (Courtesy of Dr. Susan I. Blaser.)

Table 7.3. *Classification of peroxisomal disorders.*

Defect	Some distinguishing clinical features
Disorders of peroxisomal biogenesis with multiple functional defects	
Zellweger syndrome	'Severe peroxisomal phenotype' with characteristic facial dysmorphism, disturbances of neuronal migration (polymicrogyria, neuronal heterotopias), corneal clouding, nystagmus, cataracts, congenital heart disease, poor feeding, failure to thrive, death within a few months
Neonatal adrenoleukodystrophy	'Severe peroxisomal phenotype' with more subtle facial dysmorphism, disturbances of neuronal migration (polymicrogyria, neuronal heterotopias), chemical evidence of adrenal insufficiency, poor feeding, failure to thrive, survival for up to a few years
Infantile Refsum disease	'Severe peroxisomal phenotype' with facial dysmorphism, subtle disturbances of neuronal migration (polymicrogyria, neuronal heterotopias), decreased plasma cholesterol, prominent retinal degeneration and sensorineural hearing impairment, survival for up to many years
Hyperpipecolic acidemia	'Severe peroxisomal phenotype' with prominent retinal degeneration, cirrhosis, survival for up to many years
Multiple functional defects with peroxisomes present	
Rhizomelic chondrodysplasia punctata (RCDP)	'Severe peroxisomal phenotype' with facial dysmorphism, severe shortening of proximal limbs, chondrodysplasia punctata (stippled epiphyses), skin lesions, cataracts, survival highly variable
Single enzyme defects with 'severe peroxisomal phenotype'	
DHAP acyltransferase deficiency	Identical to classical RCDP
Acyl-CoA oxidase deficiency	'Severe peroxisomal phenotype'
Bifunctional enzyme deficiency	'Severe peroxisomal phenotype' with neuronal heterotopias, polymicrogyria
3-Ketoacyl-CoA thiolase deficiency	'Severe peroxisomal phenotype' ± facial dysmorphism, renal cysts, neuronal heterotopias, early death
Dihydroxy- & trihydroxycholestanoic acidemia	'Severe peroxisomal phenotype' with subtle facial dysmorphism and liver disease, survival variable
Single enzyme defects with specific phenotype	
X-linked adrenoleukodystrophy	Rapidly progressive X-linked recessive leukodystrophy associated with adrenal insufficiency
Primary hyperoxaluria, type I	Progressive renal impairment due to renal oxalosis, nephrocalcinosis, and recurrent urolithiasis
Acatalasemia	Predisposition to certain types of bacterial infections; relatively benign

- ± impairment of special senses (visual impairment or sensorineural hearing loss).

Table 7.3 shows a classification of some of the more common peroxisomal disorders based on the nature of the basic defect. It is important not to make too much of the apparent clinical differences between various syndromes, which share so many features in common, associated with the severe peroxisomal phenotype. Ultimately, this group of disorders will be classified according to the biochemical or genetic defect as these become identified.

Rhizomelic chondrodysplasia punctata (RCDP)

RCDP is another disorder of peroxisomal function associated with severe and relatively typcial dysmorphism. Affected infants show dysmorphic facial features redolent of Zellweger syndrome, severe psychomotor retardation, profound hypotonia, cataracts, and ichthyosis. In addition, affected infants show severe shortening of proximal limbs, and the calcific stippling of epiphyses is more generalized than in Zellweger disease. Lateral radiographs of the spine typically show calcific stippling and coronal clefts of vertebral bodies.

Unlike in Zellweger syndrome and other peroxisomal disorders, plasma very long-chain fatty acid levels are normal in patients with RCDP. However, plasmalogen biosynthesis and phytanic acid oxidation are both impaired. As a result, erythocyte plasmalogen levels are decreased, and phytanic acid levels in plasma are increased, in affected infants (see Chapter 9).

Chondrodysplasia punctata (CDP) is a feature of other conditions, such as Conradi-Hünermann syndrome, an autosomal dominant condition in which limb length and intellect are normal. X-linked recessive CDP is associated with cataracts, mental retardation, and erythematous desquamative skin changes in the newborn period evolving into striated ichthyosiform hyperkeratosis within a few months. X-linked dominant CDP, a male-lethal condition, is also associated with congenital erythroderma in heterozygous females, but intellect is normal. CDP is also a feature of coumadin embryopathy.

Mitochondrial disorders

Subtle facial dysmorphism and moderately severe structural anomalies of the brain, such as congenital absence of the corpus callosum, are seen in many patients with severe variants of PDH deficiency. Facial dysmorphism and associated anomalies are much more prominent and characteristic in patients with the severe, neonatal form of glutaric aciduria type II (GA II).

Glutaric aciduria, type II

The severe hypoglycemia and metabolic acidosis in infants with the severe, neonatal form of GA II is often associated with multiple congenital anomalies, including facial dysmorphism (including high forehead, midface hypoplasia with depressed nasal bridge, hypertelorism, and low-set ears), muscular defects of the anterior abdominal wall, hypospadias, rocker-bottom feet, and cystic enlargement of the kidneys. The liver is also enlarged as a result of massive microvesicular steatosis. Abdominal ultrasound examination shows prominent cystic disease of the kidneys, and neuroimaging studies show evidence of disorganization of the cerebral cortex, a reflection of neuronal migration abnormalities.

The metabolic abnormalities generally dominate the clinical presentation, and investigation of the metabolic acidosis typically shows massive excretion of glutaric acid and other metabolites in the urine as a result of the defect in mitochondrial electron transport flavoprotein (ETF) or ETF dehydrogenase (see Chapter 4). GA II may be difficult to distinguish clinically from severe neonatal CPT II deficiency.

Biosynthetic defects

Menkes disease

Menkes disease is an X-linked recessive disorder of copper transport caused by mutations in a copper-transporting ATPase. The gene has been cloned, and many mutations have been characterized. Many of the characteristic physical abnormalities of Menkes disease are present at birth, but they may be quite subtle and are often overlooked. The face is unusual (Figure 7.9), and the skull shows abnormalities similar to those seen in patients with Zellweger syndrome: long, narrow calvarium, with high forehead and huge fontanelles; small nose, puffy eyes, hyperplastic alveolar ridges, and loose, velvety soft skin. The hair is characteristically brittle and shows pili torti on microscopic examination. Feeding problems, hypotonia, hypothermia, and diarrhea are prominent features of the disease in newborn infants. The clinical course is characterized by continued failure to thrive, profound hypotonia, intractable seizures, persistent mild normochromic normocytic anemia, chronic diarrhea, and severe developmental retardation. Survival of infants with classical severe disease rarely extends beyond two to three years.

Skeletal radiographs show generalized osteopenia and the presence of prominent wormian bones in the skull. Visualization of blood vessels reveals marked tortuosity of the arteries throughout the body. Diverticula of the bladder are common and give rise to multiple recurrent urinary tract infections. The diagnosis is suggested by finding markedly decreased copper and ceruloplasmin

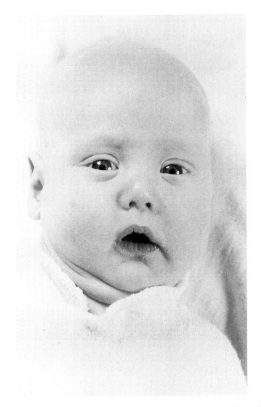

Fig. 7.9. Facial features of an infant with Menkes disease.

levels in plasma. Copper concentrations in liver are profoundly decreased; the levels in intestinal mucosa are markedly increased above normal. The copper content of cultured fibroblasts and the uptake of radioisotopic copper is greatly increased.

Treatment of the disease by daily injections of copper histidinate (about 500–1000 micrograms per day) results in normalization of plasma copper and ceruloplasmin levels. If treatment is begun within the first few days of birth, it appears to alter dramatically the course of the disease, resulting in long-term survival, freedom from seizures, and near-normal psychomotor development.

Mevalonic aciduria

Patients with mevalonic aciduria, an inborn error of cholesterol and nonsterol isoprenoid biosynthesis, present in early infancy or childhood with mildly dysmorphic facial features (Figure 7.10), severe psychomotor retardation, failure

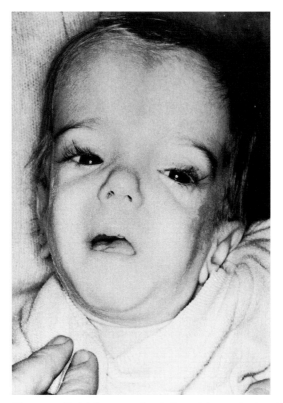

Fig. 7.10. Facial features of an infant with mevalonic aciduria. (Courtesy of Prof. Dr. G. Hoffmann, Marburg, Germany.)

to thrive, delayed closure of the cranial sutures and fontanelles, hypotonia and muscle weakness, progressive cerebellar ataxia in about half, anemia, and recurrent attacks of fever, vomiting, diarrhea, arthralgia, edema, and skin rash. In some patients, hepatosplenomegaly, lymphadenopathy, arthralgia, and uveitis during febrile crises, coupled with a dramatic response to corticosteroid treatment, might suggest a collagen vascular disease. Plasma cholesterol levels are usually normal or only slightly decreased. Creatine phosphokinase (CPK) levels are markedly elevated in the majority, particularly during febrile crises. Neuroimaging shows progressive atrophy of the cerebellar hemispheres and vermis. Urinary organic acid analysis shows high concentrations of mevalonic acid. The diagnosis is confirmed by demonstrating deficiency of mevalonate kinase in fibroblasts.

SLO syndrome

The discovery of a specific inborn error of cholesterol metabolism in patients with classical Smith-Lemli-Opitz syndrome challenged the somewhat arbitrary separation of dysmorphic syndromes from inherited metabolic diseases. It is characterized by microcephaly, failure to thrive, hypotonia, unusual facies (high forehead; cataracts; broad, short nose with anteverted nares; ptosis; micrognathia; cleft palate), limb abnormalities (syndactyly of the toes, polydactyly), genital anomalies in affected males (hypospadias, ambiguous genitalia, cryptorchidism), endocrine abnormalities, heart and kidney malformations, and psychomotor retardation. Gas chromatographic analysis of sterols shows that cholesterol levels in affected patients are decreased, and the concentration of its immediate precursor, 7-dehydrocholesterol (7-DHC), is increased in plasma, erythrocytes, and cultured skin fibroblasts. Plasma cholesterol levels measured by conventional enzymic-colorimetric analysis, which does not discriminate between cholesterol and 7-DHC, are not decreased.

Carbohydrate-deficient glycoprotein (CDG) syndrome

CDG syndrome is an uncommon autosomal recessive multisystem disease associated with an abnormality in the synthesis of circulating glycoproteins. The frequency in northern Europe is estimated to be comparable to the incidence of metachromatic leukodystrophy. It is characterized clinically by onset in early infancy of failure to thrive, marked hypotonia, severe developmental delay, particularly affecting gross motor activities, and intermittent episodes of hepatocellular dysfunction, recurrent pericadial effusions, acute encephalopathy, or stroke-like episodes. Most show facial dysmorphism with broad nasal bridge, prominent jaw and forehead, large ears, strabismus, and inverted nipples. Unusual fat pads are present over the upper, outer aspects of the buttocks, associated with thickening of the skin on the legs. Alternating areas of lipohyperplasia and lipoatrophy may occur on the thighs (Figure 7.11). The liver is enlarged and liver function tests are abnormal. In addition to marked hypotonia and generalized muscle weakness, deep tendon reflexes are initially depressed, then disappearing within two to three years.

Within three to four years, the hepatocellular and cardiac problems resolve, and the principal problems relate to the nervous system. Psychomotor development is severely impaired, and few affected children are able to walk independently. Fine motor skills are not so severely affected as gross motor abilities, and there is no regression. Ataxia and dyskinesia become more prominent. All affected children have strabismus, and develop progressive retinal degeneration. Stroke-like episodes or acute encephalopathy, seizures, and hemiparesis are

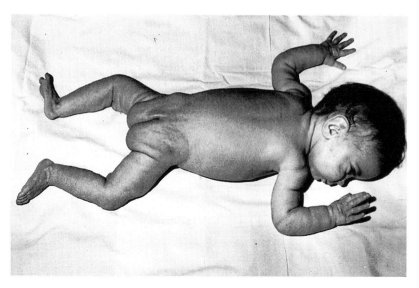

Fig. 7.11. Lipodystrophy of the buttocks and thighs of a 6-week-old infant with carbohydrate-deficient glycoprotein syndrome. (Courtesy of Prof. Dr. Jaak Jaeken, Leuven, Belgium.)

particularly common in middle childhood, usually precipitated by intercurrent febrile illnesses. As a rule these neurologic crises are followed by complete recovery.

Adolescence is characterized by marked weakness and atrophy of the muscles, particularly of the lower extremities, and slowing of nerve conduction velocities, along with continuing cerebellar ataxia and incoordination. Neuroimaging often shows cerebellar and brain stem atrophy. The chest becomes increasingly pigeon-breasted and associated with progressive thoracic kyphoscoliosis. Some patients show hypogonadism. Communication skills are characteristically more advanced than gross motor development, and affected individuals often display an almost euphoric affect. Mobility becomes increasingly compromised by the progression of flexion contractures, particularly affecting the lower extremities.

Liver function tests are generally abnormal early in the disease, but improve with age. Similarly the CSF protein is usually somewhat elevated early in the disease, becoming normal with age; however, in some patients, the CSF protein increases with age. Affected individuals have subnormal levels of various plasma glycoproteins: thryoxine-binding globulin, haptoglobin, transcortin, apolipoprotein B and low density lipoprotein (LDL)-cholesterol, and coagulation factors. The most characteristic biochemical finding is a pronounced abnormality of the

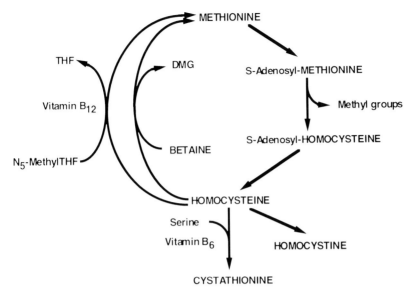

Fig. 7.12. Metabolism of homocysteine and methionine.
Abbreviations: N5-methylTHF, N5-methyltetrahydrofolate; THF, tetrahydrofolate;
DMG, N,N-dimethylglycine.

N-linked oligosaccharides of circulating glycoproteins, especially transferrin.
Typically, the terminal trisaccharides of many of the glycoprotein oligosaccharides are missing. Demonstration of the abnormality requires electrofocusing
analysis of the glycoprotein; the levels of transferrin as measured by conventional
immunochemical techniques are generally normal. The underlying defect in the
type I variant of the disease is deficiency of phosphomannomutase.

Homocystinuria
Marked accumulation of homocystine (a dimer of homocysteine), irrespective of
the underlying cause, is associated with certain dysmorphic features arising, in
part, as a result of the effects of the amino acid on the levels and cross-linking of
various connective tissue elements. Homocysteine is an intermediate in the
biosynthesis of methionine and cystathionine (Figure 7.12). Accumulation
occurs as a result of defects in any of a number of reactions (Table 7.4), including
several involving the metabolism of vitamin B_{12}, an obligatory cofactor for
methionine synthase activity (see Figure 4.5). The commonest cause of
homocystinuria/hyperhomocyst(e)inemia, and that associated with the most
severe accumulation of the amino acids, is *cystathionine β-synthase* (CBS)
deficiency.

Table 7.4. *Genetic and some acquired causes of homocystinuria/hyperhomocyst(e)*
inemia

Impaired cystathionine β-synthase (CBS) activity
Genetic CBS deficiency
Some drugs (e.g., 6-azauridine triacetate)

Impaired methionine synthase activity
Genetic tetrahydrofolate reductase deficiency
Genetic failure of vitamin B_{12} absorption (Immerslund syndrome)
Impaired cellular uptake of B_{12} (Transcobalamin II deficiency)
Impaired release of B_{12} from lysosomes (*cblF*)
Impaired conversion of B_{12} to methyl- or adenosyl-B_{12} (*cblC* and *cblD*)
Impaired conversion of B_{12} to methyl-B_{12} (*cblE* or *cblG*)
Nutritional B_{12} deficiency
Nutritional folate deficiency

Note: Adapted from Mudd *et al.* (1995).

Homocystinuria due to genetic deficiency of CBS is characterized by
moderately severe mental retardation, connective tissue abnormalities affecting
the skeleton and eyes, vascular abnormalities, and other less prominent physical
anomalies. Affected children usually come to initial medical attention in the first
one to two years of life as a result of developmental retardation. The
psychomotor development of untreated patients varies tremendously; most
remain moderately retarded. Seizures may also occur. Psychiatric and behavioral
problems are common, but frank psychosis is rare.

One of the most consistent and prominent physical abnormalities in
CBS-deficiency homocystinuria is dislocation of the ocular lens. Dislocation is
downward, as opposed to the upward dislocation of the lens in Marfan
syndrome, and it generally occurs between 4 and 12 years of age. Some patients
escape this complication until the third decade of life. The parents may be the
first to notice the shimmering iridodonesis of the iris, a quivering movement of
the membrane usually precipitated by movement of the head. Dislocation is
associated with the development of marked myopia, and spontaneous retinal
detachment is common. Less commonly, it is associated with glaucoma,
cataracts, retinal degeneration, and optic atrophy.

Osteoporosis is also a prominent feature of the disease by the late teens, most
commonly affecting the spine. It is often associated with the development of
thoracic scoliosis. Abnormal lengthening of the long bones (dolichostenomelia)
causes affected individuals to be very tall and lean by the time they reach late

adolescence. Pectus carinatum, pes cavus, genu valgum, and radiologic abnormalities of the vertebrae are common. Although the body habitus is marfanoid, affected patients do not have true arachnodactyly, hypermobility of joints, or the cardiac abnormalities of Marfan syndrome.

Thromboembolism is the most frequent cause of death of individuals with CBS-deficiency homocystinuria. The most common site of intravascular thrombosis is peripheral veins, setting the stage for embolization to the lungs. Cerebrovascular, peripheral arterial, and coronary artery thrombosis also occur. Thromboembolism may occur at any age, even in infants with the disease. However, the likelihood of clinically significant problems increases with age, the cumulative risk reaching 25% by age 15–20 years.

In about half the patients with CBS-deficiency homocystinuria, the biochemical abnormalities are normalized by treatment with large doses (250–500 mg per day) of pyridoxine. In general, the extent and severity of the complications of the disease, including thromboembolism, are greater in patients who are unresponsive to vitamin therapy.

What sort of metabolic studies are most likely to be diagnostically productive in the investigation of dysmorphism?

If disorders of organelle metabolism are major contributors to those inherited metabolic diseases associated with dysmorphism, it follows that investigation aimed at assessing oganelle function would be particularly important to establishing a diagnosis. In order to be able to concentrate here on general principles, much of the detail relating to the investigation of organelle function is discussed later in Chapter 9.

Morphologic studies are often helpful in the assessment of possible disorders of organelle function. Non-invasive imaging studies (ultrasound examination, plain radiographs, CT scanning, and MRI studies) help to establish the pattern and degree of involvement of various organs and tissues. Sometimes the type and pattern of abnormalities are characteristic enough to suggest a specific diagnosis. More often, the abnormalities may suggest a class of disorders, such as lysosomal storage diseases, but are not specific enough to pin the diagnosis down to a specific inborn error of metabolism. For example, finding generalized dysostosis multiplex on plain radiographs is a strong indication of a lysosomal storage disorder. Similarly, the presence of CT or MRI evidence of cerebral cortical disorganization is typical, though not diagnostic, of some peroxisomal disorders. Confirmation of a metabolic diagnosis invariably requires specific biochemical studies.

Table 7.5. *Initial metabolic investigation of patients presenting with storage syndrome or dysmorphism.*

Urinary mucopolysaccharide screening test
Urinary oligosaccharide screening test
Urinary organic acid analysis
Plasma lactate and pyruvate
Plasma very long-chain fatty acids
Plasma phytanic acid
Plasma amino acid analysis

Unlike disorders of small molecule metabolism, in which histopathologic changes are generally not very helpful, inborn errors of organelle function are commonly associated with histopathologic and ultrastructural abnormalities which are sufficiently characteristic to suggest a short list of diagnostic possibilities. For example, the histopathologic and histochemical characteristics of the storage histiocytes in subcutaneous granulomas in patients with Farber lipogranulomatosis are virtually pathognomonic of the disease. The absence of normal peroxisomes in the liver is characteristic of severe peroxisomal assembly defects, like Zellweger syndrome. The increased number and abnormal structure of the mitochondria in skeletal muscle is highly suggestive of a mitochondrial ETC defect, though which subunit or complex is involved would require further studies.

The types of biochemical studies needed ultimately to arrive at a diagnosis include tests directed primarily at organelle-classification of a disorder (Table 7.5) and tests for specific defects. If the results of any of these are abnormal, further studies would be needed to identify a specific enzyme defect.

The approach to the identification of dysmorphism arising as a result of defects in biosynthesis, such as CDG syndrome, is not nearly so direct. In fact, the recommendation of any particular test to screen for inborn errors of biosynthesis would obviously omit some of the known and most of the currently unknown defects in biosynthesis presenting with dysmorphic features. Instead, the approach to be encouraged is one of intellectual receptivity. That is to say, the clinician should approach the metabolic investigation of a dysmorphic patient with the commitment to explain *every* laboratory abnormality that comes to light. This is contrary to the general tendancy to ignore or dismiss any information, particularly from the laboratory, which does not fit the presumptive clinical diagnosis. This is a particularly difficult group of diseases to manage: there are no 'screening tests' for inborn errors of biosynthesis.

Bibliography

Clayton, P.T. & Thompson, E. (1988). Dysmorphic syndromes with demonstrable biochemical abnormalities. *Journal of Medical Genetics*, **25**, 463–72.

Jaeken, J., Stibler, H. & Hagberg, B. (Eds.) (1991). The carbohydrate-deficient glycoprotein syndrome. *Acta Paediatrica Scandinavica*, Supplement 375, 5–71.

Jones, K.L. (1988). *Smith's Recognizable Patterns of Human Malformation*, 4th edn. Philadelphia: W.B. Saunders Company.

Lowden, J.A. (1981). Approaches to the diagnosis and management of infants and children with lysosomal storage diseases. In *Genetic Issues in Pediatric and Obstetric Practice*, ed. M.M. Kaback, pp. 267–305. Chicago: Year Book Publishers, Inc.

Moser, A.B., Rasmussen, M., Naidu, S., Watkins, P.A., McGuinness, M., Hajra, A., Chen, G., Raymond, G., Liu, A., Gordon, D., Garnaas, K., Walton, D.S., Skjeldal, O.H., Guggenheim, M.A., Jackson, L.G., Elias, E.R. & Moser, H.W. (1995). Phenotype of patients with peroxisomal disorders subdivided into sixteen complementation groups. *Journal of Pediatrics*, **127**, 13–22.

Mudd, H., Levy, H.L. & Skovby, F. (1995). Disorders of transsulfuration. In *The Metabolic and Molecular Bases of Inherited Disease*, 7th edn., ed. C.R. Scriver, A.L. Beaudet, W.S. Sly & D. Valle, pp. 1279–327. New York: McGraw-Hill.

Poggi-Travert, F., Fournier, B., Poll-The, B.T. & Saudubray, J.-M. (1995). Clincial approach to inherited peroxisomal disorders. In *Diagnosis of Human Peroxisomal Disorders*, ed. F. Roels, S. DeBie, R.B.H. Schutgens & G.T.N. Besley, pp. 1–18. Dordrecht: Kluwer Academic Publishers.

Wanders, R.J.A., Schutgens, R.B.H. & Barth, P.G. (1995). Peroxisomal disorders: a review. *Journal of Neuropathology and Experimental Neurology*, **54**, 726–39.

8

Acute metabolic illness in the newborn

There are few situations in medicine as acutely stressful as the precipitate deterioration of a previously healthy newborn infant, coupled with the recognition that, irrespective of the cause, delay in recognition and initiation of appropriate management often leads to death or irreparable brain damage. Severe illness in the newborn, regardless of the underlying cause, tends to manifest itself in a rather stereotypic way with relatively nonspecific findings, such as poor feeding, drowsiness, lethargy, hypotonia, and failure to thrive. Because inherited metabolic diseases are individually rare, clinicians have a tendancy to pursue the possibility only after other more common conditions, such as sepsis, have been excluded. Further delay often occurs because the type of investigation required to make the diagnosis of inherited metabolic disease includes unfamiliar tests, which the clinician may feel uncomfortable interpreting owing to a general lack of confidence regarding metabolic problems.

The need for despatch requires that inborn errors of metabolism be considered *along with and at the same time as* common acquired conditions, such as sepsis, hypoxic-ischemic encephalopathy, intraventricular hemorrhage, intoxications, congenital viral infections, and certain types of congenital heart disease. Appropriate laboratory investigation, including some simple bedside tests, such as urine tests for reducing substances and ketones, should be initiated without delay, even done at the bedside if possible. Despite the apparent nonspecificity of presenting symptoms in neonates with inherited metabolic diseases, there are some features which increase the likelihood of an inborn error of metabolism.

Suspicion

A history of acute deterioration after a period of apparent normalcy, which may be as short as a few hours, is a feature of many inherited metabolic diseases presenting in the newborn period. This is particularly true of inborn errors of metabolism in which symptoms are caused by postnatal accumulation of toxic, low molecular weight metabolites, which had been removed prenatally by

176

diffusion across the placenta and metabolism by the mother. Conditions in which this occurs include some of the amino acidopathies (notably nonketotic hyperglycinemia, maple syrup urine disease (MSUD), and hepatorenal tyrosinemia), urea cycle enzyme defects, many of the organic acidopathies, galactosemia, and hereditary fructose intolerance. Although a period of apparent normalcy is a frequent characteristic of these disorders, its absence does not exclude them from consideration. It may be obscured by coincident neonatal problems, such as birth trauma or complications of prematurity.

Along with a history of acute deterioration after a period of apparent normalcy, a family history of a similar illness in a sibling or other blood relative, or a history of parental consanguinity, increases the possibility of an inherited metabolic disease.

Prominent nonspecific signs of diffuse cerebral dysfunction, especially if they are progressive, are a strong indication of inherited metabolic disease. The onset is usually gradual, often no more than poor sucking, drowsiness, and some floppiness. The mother may notice a change in the baby which is often initially dismissed by medical attendants. Vomiting often occurs, and it may be severe enough to suggest mechanical bowel obstruction. Deterioration is marked by increasing somnolence, progressing to stupor and coma, associated with the development of abnormalities of tone (hypotonia or hypertonia) and posturing (fisting, opisthotonus), abnormal movements (tongue-thrusting, lip-smacking, bicycling, tonic elevation of the arms, coarse tremors, myoclonic jerks), and disturbances of breathing (periodic respiration, tachypnea, apneic spells, hic-coughing), bradycardia, and hypothermia. Early in the course of the deterioration, the signs of encephalopathy often fluctuate with periods of what might seem like improvement alternating with periods of obvious progression, or periods of hypotonia punctuated by episodes of hypertonia, tremulousness, posturing, and myoclonus. The EEG generally shows nonspecific encephalopathic changes, often progressing to a burst-suppression pattern indicative of severe diffuse encephalopathy.

Much has been made of the importance of unusual odors in the early recognition of the possibility of an inborn error of metabolism. However, with the exception of MSUD, these odors are rarely prominent or characteristic enough in newborn infants to be diagnostically useful. In fact, unusual dietary preferences of mothers appears to be a more common cause of abnormal odors in breast-fed infants. Signs specifically attributable to inherited metabolic diseases are sometimes obscured by problems commonly associated with acquired diseases. For example, organic acidopathies presenting in the newborn period are commonly associated with neutropenia, and sepsis often occurs in these patients as a result of the increased susceptibility to bacterial infection. The encephalopathy and metabolic acidosis caused by the metabolic disorder may be wrongly attributed entirely to the septicemia. The recognition of subtle clinical discrepancies between the severity of the apparent sepsis and the degree of acidosis in this situation may make the difference between early diagnosis of an inborn error of organic acid metabolism and missing it completely. There are some apparently acquired conditions in the newborn which are particularly common complications of inherited metabolic diseases. For example, *Escherichia coli* sepsis is common in infants with classical galactosemia. Pulmonary hemorrhage or primary respiratory alkalosis may be important clinical clues to hyperammonemia caused by a urea cycle enzyme defect (UCED).

Initial laboratory investigation

It is impossible to exaggerate the importance of speed in the invetigation and treatment of possible inborn errors of metabolism in the newborn. *Metabolic investigations should be initiated as soon as the possibility is considered, not after all other explanations for illness have been eliminated.* This is particularly important for those conditions associated with hyperammonemia, such as the UCEDs, transient hyperammonemia of the newborn, and the organic acidopathies. The outcome of treatment of these disorders is directly related to the rapidity with which metabolic problems are suspected and appropriate basic medical management is initiated.

An outline of the initial laboratory investigation of suspected inherited metabolic disease in an acutely ill infant or child is presented in Table 8.1.

Some laboratory studies undertaken in the course of the investigation of other causes of disease are also helpful in the identification of possible inborn errors of metabolism. For example, plasma electrolyte abnormalities, identified in the course of the management of a newborn in shock of obscure etiology, may suggest adrenogenital syndrome. The routine urinalysis may be very helpful in the initial investigation of a newborn infant presenting with an acute encephalopathy due to MSUD: the urine often tests strongly for ketones, something in the newborn that should always be considered abnormal and investigated further. Similarly, the presence of marked neutropenia and thrombocytopenia in a newborn infant with clinical evidence of an encephalopathy and acute metabolic acidosis may signal a diagnosis of methylmalonic acidemia or propionic acidemia. The measurement of blood gases and plasma electrolytes and glucose is so widespread in acute-care pediatrics that a severe persistent metabolic acidosis would not likely be missed in an acutely ill infant. The measurement of blood ammonia should be carried out at the first indication of

Table 8.1. *Initial laboratory investigation of suspected inherited metabolic disease presenting in the newborn period.*

Blood	Hemoglobin, white blood count, platelets
	Blood gases and plasma electrolytes (calculate anion gap)
	Glucose
	Ammonium
	Lactate
	Calcium and magnesium
	Liver function tests, including albumin and prothrombin and partial thromboplastin times
	Amino acid analysis QUANTITATIVE
	Carnitine, total and free
	Galactosemia screening test
	Plasma for storage at –20°C: 2–5 ml
Urine	Ketones (Ames Acetest)
	Reducing substances (Ames Clinitest)
	Ketoacids (DNPH)
	Sulfites (Merck Sulfitest)
	Organic acids (GC–MS)
	Urine for storage at –20°C: 10–20 ml

Note: Abbreviations: DNPH, dinitrophenylhydrazine; GC–MS, gas chromatography-mass spectrometry.

trouble, at the same time one might consider measuring the blood glucose, gases, and electrolytes in a seriously sick newborn.

The importance of the analysis of plasma amino acids and urinary organic acids in the diagnosis of inborn errors of amino acid metabolism is widely accepted. It is imperative that the analysis of plasma amino acids should be *quantitative* and carried out early in the investigation of any acutely ill infant in whom the possibility of an inborn error of metabolism is suspected. While it is somewhat more labor intensive than screening chromatography, quantitative analysis of amino acids in plasma is faster, and it is of critical importance in the diagnosis of specific amino acidopathies and in the differential diagnosis of hyperammonemia. By contrast, quantitative analysis of amino acids in urine in the newborn period is rarely immediately helpful.

Analysis of urinary organic acids by gas chromatography–mass spectrometry is critical to the early diagnosis of a number of treatable inborn errors of metabolism, such as methylmalonic acidemia, propionic acidemia, and defects in fatty acid oxidation. The technical issues are discussed in detail in Chapter 9. The results are often diagnostic, even in the absence of any other biochemical

Table 8.2. *Inherited metabolic disorders presenting in the newborn period with acute encephalopathy without metabolic acidosis.*

Disorder	Distinguishing features
Maple syrup urine disease	Plasma ammonium normal; urine positive for ketones; urinary DNPH test positive; marked elevation of plasma branched chain amino acids
Urea cycle enzyme defects	Plasma ammonium >250 μmol/L in absence of metabolic acidosis; normal liver function tests
Nonketotic hyperglycinemia	Elevated CSF glycine; no acidosis; no hyperammonemia; no hypoglycemia
Pyridoxine-dependent seizures	Therapeutic trial of vitamin B_6
Peroxisomal disorders (Zellweger syndrome)	Dysmorphism (see Chpater 7); elevated plasma very long chain fatty acids
Molybdenum cofactor defect	Sulfites increased in urine; plasma urate levels low; increased S-sulfocysteine in urine

Note: Abbreviations: DNPH, dinitrophenylhydrazine; CSF, cerebrospinal fluid.

abnormality. Analysis of urinary organic acids should, therefore, be considered early in the investigation of a possible inherited metabolic disease. Organic acid analysis, including analysis of organic acid esters, requires only 5–10 ml of urine. If analysis is delayed, the urine should be stored and transported frozen at –20°C or lower. Under these conditions, most diagnostically important organic acids in urine are stable for several days to weeks.

Although the presence of nonglucose reducing substances in the urine of a sick newborn may suggest galactosemia, their absence does not rule out the possibility. Even short-term galactose restriction is usually sufficient to reverse the galactosuria of the disease. Because the enzyme defect is demonstrable in erythrocytes, but not plasma, specimens of whole blood should be submitted for galactosemia screening, and the blood must be obtained before the infant receives any transfused blood.

Four clinical 'syndromes'

There are very few pathognomonic clinical signs that permit the immediate clinical diagnosis of inborn errors of metabolism in the newborn period. However, like inherited metabolic diseases presenting later in life, those with onset in the newborn period commonly describe one of four 'syndromes': (1) encephalopathy without metabolic acidosis; (2) encephalopathy with metabolic acidosis; (3) hepatic syndrome; or (4) non-immune fetal hydrops. Some of these disorders are associated with dysmorphic features which are discussed in Chapter 7.

Encephalopathy without metabolic acidosis

Encephalopathy without metabolic acidosis is a common problem in neonatology, most often the result of an hypoxic-ischemic insult to the brain occurring at or shortly after birth. A history of a period of apparent normalcy, or the absence of a history of birth trauma in keeping with the degree of encephalopathy, should be treated as indicators of the possibility of an inborn error of metabolism. There are six inherited metabolic diseases which characteristically present in the newborn period in this way (Table 8.2).

Maple syrup urine disease (MSUD)

MSUD is caused by a defect in branched-chain amino acid metabolism characterized by deficiency of the enzyme, α-ketoacyl-CoA decarboxylase, which catalyzes the second step in the oxidative metabolism of leucine, isoleucine, and valine. The defect causes accumulation of the respective 2-ketoacids and the branched-chain amino acids. Affected infants commonly present in the second or third week of life, though we have infants who presented with encephalopathy as early as within the first 24 hours of life. The clinical findings are of a progressive, nonspecific, acute encephalopathy. The diagnosis can sometimes be made at the bedside owing to the peculiar odor associated with the disease and the positive test for ketones in the urine. Although the disease received its name from the alleged resemblance of the smell to that of maple syrup, the odor actually more closely resembles that of burnt sugar, which should be a relief to clinicians who do not have access to the syrup, a product almost exclusively of eastern Canada and northeastern US. Severe, intractible cerebral edema causing massive intracranial hypertension, with bulging fontanelle and diastasis of the sutures, develops relatively early and is invariably an indication of a poor prognosis. Although hypoglycemia has been reported in newborn infants with MSUD, this is a rare phenomenon in our experience. Although severe abnormalities of tone (hypotonia and hypertonia), posturing, and abnormal neurovegetative movement are prominent in infants with advanced leucine encephalopathy, frank seizures only occur late in the disorder.

Although the urine of infants with MSUD generally tests strongly positive for ketones, metabolic acidosis is *not* a prominent finding until late in the course of the disease. This is important. The encephalopathy of MSUD is apparently caused by accumulation of leucine, not by accumulation of the 2-ketoacids. The diagnosis is confirmed by quantitative analysis of plasma amino acids. Analysis of urinary organic acids as oxime derivatives (Chapter 9) shows the presence of branched-chain 2-ketoacids and 2-hydroxyacids. Modest elevations of plasma branched-chain amino acids are commonly seen in infants and children after short-term starvation; the levels in MSUD presenting in the newborn period are several times higher.

Treatment requires aggressive measures to lower plasma leucine levels, invariably including some form of efficient dialysis, such as hemodialysis or continuous venous–venous hemofiltration-dialysis (CVVHD). Intravenous lipid, along with high concentrations of glucose, is administered in an effort to decrease endogenous protein breakdown. Insulin is sometimes given, along with sufficient glucose to prevent hypoglycemia, in an attempt to increase endogenous protein biosynthesis. The clinical effectiveness of insulin in this situation is still not proven. The administration of mannitol, or other measures to try to control the cerebral edema, is not generally effective.

Urea cycle enzyme defects (UCED)

The metabolism of ammonium is reviewed in some detail in Chapter 2. Some of the defects presenting as hyperammonemic encephalopathy in older children or

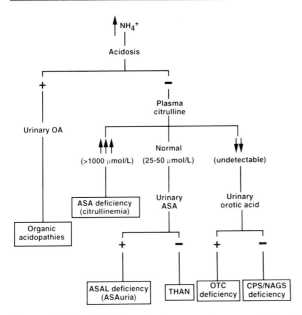

Fig. 8.1. Differential diagnosis of urea cycle enzyme defects in the newborn. Abbreviations: OA, organic acids; ASA, argininosuccinic acid synthetase; ASAL, argininosuccinic acid lyase; THAN, transient hyperammonemia of the newborn; OTC, ornithine transcarbamylase; CPS, carbamylphosphate synthetase I; NAGS, N-acetylglutamate synthetase.

adults do not cause symptomatic hyperammonemia in the newborn period. The differential diagnosis of neonatal hyperammonemic encephalopathy lends itself well to an algorithmic approach (Figure 8.1), initially proposed by Saul Brusilow and his colleagues at Johns Hopkins Medical Center.

The onset and early course of the acute encephalopathy in infants with UCED is similar to that in MSUD, though hypotonia is more prominent and severe, and breathing may be abnormally rapid producing respiratory alkalosis as a result of stimulation of ventilation by ammonium. Having determined the presence of significant hyperammonemia (>250 μmol/L; often as high as 2000 μmol/L), measurement of blood gases and plasma electrolytes shows whether ammonium accumulation is likely due to a UCED or is secondary to an organic acidopathy. The degree of the hyperammonemia is of no help in this regard: infants with organic acidopathies or with transient hyperammonemia of the newborn (THAN) will often have plasma ammonium levels at presentation in the same range as infants with untreated UCED.

The UCEDs presenting in the newborn period are clinically indistinguishable from each other. Differential diagnosis rests critically on quantitative analysis of plasma amino acids. The citrulline level is particularly important, though normal levels in newborn infants are so low that some laboratories do not calculate the concentration unless it is specifically requested. Very high citrulline levels indicate the UCED is citrullinemia caused by deficiency of argininosuccinic acid (ASA) synthetase. Abnormally low citrulline levels suggest a defect in citrulline production, as a result of deficiency of either ornithine transcarbamylase (OTC) or carbamylphosphate synthetase I (CPS I). OTC deficiency is the most common of the UCEDs, and it is the only one transmitted as an X-linked recessive disorder. Although heterozygous females often present later in infancy or childhood, they almost never present with hyperammonemic encephalopathy in the newborn period. OTC deficiency is characterized by accumulation of carbamylphosphate, an intermediate in cytosolic pyrimidine biosynthesis. Diffusion of the compound from mitochondria into the cytosol stimulates pyrimidine biosynthesis causing accumulation of orotic acid. The presence of increased concentrations of orotic acid in the urine distinguishes OTC deficiency from CPS deficiency.

Normal or only modestly elevated plasma citrulline levels are seen in ASA lyase deficiency and in infants with THAN, which is often clinically distinguishable from ASA lyase deficiency and the other UCEDs. It is not an inherited metabolic disease. It is a condition of unknown etiology, generally affecting premature infants, usually with a history of low birth weight and respiratory distress. It also usually presents within the first 24 hours of life, unlike the UCED, which commonly present on or after the third day of life. The presence of ASA and its anhydrides in plasma, which is seen on the same quantitative amino acid analysis used to measure citrulline, confirms the diagnosis of ASA lyase deficiency. Infants with ASA lyase deficiency also have very low plasma arginine levels. This is therapeutically important. The hyperammonemia in infants with ASA lyase deficiency is caused by inadequacy of the supply of ornithine, derived from arginine, to combine with the carbamylphosphate produced from condensation of ammonium and bicarbonate. In a sense, therefore, the hyperammonemia is the result of secondary CPS I deficiency. Treatment of affected infants with intravenous arginine produces dramatic resolution of the hyperammonemia over a period of only a few hours, a response that is so typical that it is diagnostic of the disease.

The successful treatment of hyperammonemic encephalopathy caused by UCED demands early and very aggressive measures to control ammonium production and facilitate its elimination. Intravenous glucose and lipid minimize ammonium production from endogenous protein breakdown. The administration of arginine is recommended even before the specific UCED has been identified because the amino acid is dramatically beneficial in patients with ASA lyase deficiency, at least modestly beneficial in the others, except perhaps in ASA synthetase deficiency, and harmful in none. The intravenous administration of sodium benzoate and sodium phenylacetate (or sodium phenylbutyrate, which is converted to sodium phenylacetate in the body) is used extensively in the treatment of neonatal hyperammonemia, including that associated with UCED. These compounds lower ammonium levels by facilitating waste nitrogen excretion by alternative pathways (see Chapter 10). Specifically, sodium benzoate condenses with glycine to form hippuric acid, which is cleared from the circulation very efficiently by the kidney. Each molecule of benzoate metabolized in this fashion causes excretion of one atom of nitrogen. Sodium phenylacetate condenses with glutamine to form phenylacetylglutamine, which is also excreted in the urine taking with it two atoms of nitrogen per molecule. Since both glycine and glutamine are nonessential amino acids, they perform in this therapeutic strategy as a waste nitrogen 'metabolic sponge'.

Except in infants with ASA lyase deficiency, who respond so well to intravenous arginine, ammonium levels during acute hyperammonemia cannot be controlled adequately by medical measures alone. Restoration of normal plasma ammonium levels requires some form of aggressive dialysis, either hemodialysis or CVVHD. Regrettably, although the prognosis for infants with THAN who are identified and treated early and aggressively is excellent, the mortality associated with the disorder is over 50% in most centers owing primarily to delayed diagnosis.

Nonketotic hyperglycinemia (NKHG)
NKHG, due to deficiency of the hepatic glycine cleavage reaction, is characterized by early onset, rapidly progressive encephalopathy with virtually no secondary biochemical abnormalities to provide a clue to the underlying defect. In fact, it is the lack of acidosis, ketosis, hypoglycemia, hyperammonemia, hepatocellular dysfunction, cardiac, renal, or hematologic abnormalities, in the face of clinical evidence of very severe diffuse cerebral dysfunction, which suggests the diagnosis. The encephalopathy characteristically progresses quickly to respiratory arrest, and many affected infants become intubated and ventilated before the diagnosis is confirmed.

Analysis of plasma amino acids usually shows elevation of glycine concentrations. However, plasma concentrations may be only modestly elevated in affected infants, and sometimes they are normal, presumably because glycine reabsorption by the kidney is not mature at birth. Renal clearances of the amino acid are high, and urinary glycine levels are almost always elevated. Since elevations of plasma glycine are a common manifestation of various disorders of organic acid metabolism, hyperglycinemia by itself is not sufficient to make the diagnosis. The elevation of glycine levels in the cerebrospinal fluid (CSF) is sufficiently consistent and specific to be considered diagnostic of the disease.

Treatment of NKHG is unsatisfactory. Aggressive treatment with intravenous fluids, glucose, and sodium benzoate will restore plasma glycine levels to normal, or even much lower. However, treatment has little effect on CSF glycine levels. Attempts have been made to treat the condition with neuromodulators, such as diazepam, strychnine, and, more recently, with dextromethorphan. Only dextromethorphan appears to have any beneficial effect, and the effect is incomplete. Curiously, after several days of ventilatory support, infants with NKHG often appear to improve and can be safely extubated. However, almost all will have suffered very severe, irreparable brain damage. A small number of cases has been reported in which the defect in glycine metabolism appears to be severe, but transient. Most of the patients with this rare, transient variant of the disease are currently alive and apparently well.

Pyridoxine-dependent seizures

Pyridoxine-dependent seizures is one of the few inherited metabolic diseases in which seizures are particularly prominent and severe in the absence of any other significant clinical abnormality (see Chapter 2). Affected infants characteristically present very early, in the first few hours or days of life, with intractible, generalized, tonic-clonic seizures and associated EEG abnormalities. On direct questionning, the mother of the infant will often report that she was aware of paroxysms of fetal movement later in the course of the pregnancy. These have been interpreted to be intrauterine convulsions. Apart from the seizures, affected infants appear normal, though failure to control the convulsions invariably results in the ultimate development of moderately severe mental retardation. The most remarkable feature of this condition, which may be the result of a defect in glutamic acid decarboxylase, is its dramatic response to administration of vitamin B_6 (pyridoxine). The intravenous administration of 100 mg of the vitamin results in prompt cessation of the seizures and normalization of the EEG abnormalities.

Peroxisomal disorders (Zellweger syndrome)

Infants with Zellweger syndrome are often acutely symptomatic within a few hours of birth. They characteristically show profound hypotonia, typical abnormalities of the face and skull, nystagmus, seizures, jaundice, hepatomegaly, and other anomalies which are described in more detail in Chapter 7. Plain radiographs of the long bones shows the presence of abnormal punctate califications in the epiphyses of the knees and other joints; ultrasound examination of the abdomen shows enlargement of the liver and kidneys with cystic changes in both organs; and CT scans of the head show cerebral dysgenesis with subcortical cystic changes. Routine laboratory studies show evidence of hepatocellular dysfunction with elevated of bilirubin and transaminases, hypoalbuminemia, and prolonged prothrombin and partial thromboplastic times. Confirmatory biochemical abnormalities specific to the disease include elevation of plasma levels of very long-chain fatty acids (C26:0 and C26:1), decreased erythrocyte plasmalogens, and the presence of pipecolic acid and bile acid intermediates in plasma. Liver biopsy shows evidence of bile stasis, cystic changes, and fibrosis; electron microscopic examination reveals the absence of peroxisomes.

Molybdenum cofactor deficiency (sulfite oxidase/xanthine oxidase deficiency)
The development, within the first week or two of birth, of intractible tonic-clonic seizures in an encephalopathic infant without hypoglycemia, hypocalcemia, hyperammonemia, or significant metabolic acidosis, is suggestive of molybdenum cofactor deficiency, or the rarer disorder, isolated sulfite oxidase deficiency. Imaging studies may show early cerebral edema followed rapidly by marked cerebral and cerebellar atrophy, hydrocephalus *ex vacuo*, and signs of hypomyelination of white matter. The presence of evidence of cerebral dysgenesis suggests that considerable damage occurs before birth.

Molybdenum cofactor deficiency is associated with combined deficiency of the two molybdenum-dependent enzymes, xanthine oxidase and sulfite oxidase. The clinical and pathologic abnormalities in isolated sulfite oxidase deficiency are indistinguishable from the changes in molybdenum cofactor deficiency. The deficiency of xanthine oxidase causes marked depression of plasma uric acid levels, an important and easily accessible clue to the underlying disorder. Urine amino acid analysis shows the presence of increased levels of S-sulfocysteine. However, the diagnosis can often be made at the bedside by tests of the urine for the presence of sulfite using commercially available dipsticks (Merckoquant 10013 Sulfit Test). The urine must be fresh because sulfite is oxidized rapidly in air at room temperature. The disease is almost always associated with severe brain damage and death in early childhood. Survival beyond two years of age is often, though not always, associated with the development of dislocation of the ocular lens.

Encephalopathy with metabolic acidosis

In infants with inherited metabolic diseases characterized by encephalopathy associated with metabolic acidosis, the tachypnea associated with the acidosis may be severe enough to suggest a diagnosis of primary pulmonary disease. Typically, the infant is apparently well until three to five days of age when feeding difficulties and other nonspecific signs of encephalopathy develop, accompanied by a significant increase in respiratory rate and effort. Chest radiographs typically show nothing more sinister than some hyperinflation, and the measurement of blood gases confirms the presence of a primary metabolic acidosis.

The diagnostic workup is similar to that described in more detail in Chapter 4. Metabolic acidosis due to renal tubular bicarbonate losses, severe enough to be clinically obvious, is rare in newborn infants; by comparison, metabolic acidosis caused by accumulation of organic acids is relatively common. The anion gap in these patients is usually increased (>25 mmol/L), and measurement of lactate, 3-hydroxybutyrate, and acetoacetate usually account for only part of the increase. *Identification of the unmeasured anion by urinary organic acid analysis is an important lead to making a diagnosis.*

Organic acidurias

Although many of the disorders of organic acid metabolism presenting later in infancy or childhood (Chapter 4) may present in the newborn period, some are relatively common and are particularly likely to present in the first few weeks of life, rather than later (Table 8.3).

Propionic acidemia, methylmalonic acidemia, and *isovaleric acidemia,* are almost clinically indistinguishable from each other when they present as acute illness in the newborn period. In each, metabolic decompensation is heralded by signs of encephalopathy accompanied by marked metabolic acidosis. In isovaleric acidemia, it is often associated with a peculiar odor. Hyperammonemia is common, and it is often severe ($NH_4^+ > 1000$ μmol/L). Neutropenia and thrombocytopenia also occur, predisposing affected infants to bacterial infection and bleeding. Plasma carnitine levels are decreased, and the proportion of esterified carnitine, relative to total carnitine (normally approximately 0.25), is generally markedly increased. Plasma amino acid analysis shows marked increases in glycine concentrations. Tests for ketones in the urine are often positive. Urinary organic acid analysis shows changes typical of the various disorders. In some centers rapid and specific diagnosis is possible by mass spectrometric (MS) analysis of plasma acylcarnitines (see Chapter 9). Confirmation of the diagnosis requires analysis of the relevant enzyme activities in cultured skin fibroblasts, coupled in some cases with specific mutation analysis.

Table 8.3. *Organic acidopathies presenting as acute illness in the newborn period.*

Disease	Defect	Urinary organic acids	Distinguishing features
Propionic acidemia	Propionyl-CoA carboxylase	Propionate, 3-hydroxypropionate, methylcitrate, propionylglycine, tiglylglycine, 3-hydroxybutyrate, acetoacetate	Severe metabolic acidosis, hyperammonemia, neutropenia, thrombocytopenia
Methylmalonic acidemia	Methylmalonyl-CoA mutase; *Cbl* defects, especially *A* and *B*	Methylmalonate, methylcitrate, 3-hydroxybutyrate, acetoacetate	Severe metabolic acidosis, hyperammonemia, neutropenia, thrombocytopenia
Isovaleric acidemia	Isovaleryl-CoA dehydrogenase	Isovalerylglycine, 3-hydroxyisovalerate, lactate, 3-hydroxybutyrate, acetoacetate	Severe metabolic acidosis, hyperammonemia, neutropenia, thrombocytopenia, odor of sweaty feet
Holocarboxylase synthetase deficiency	Holocarboxylase synthetase	Lactate, 3-hydroxybutyrate and acetoacetate (due to PC deficiency); 3-methylcrotonate, 3-methylcrotonylglycine, 3-hydroxyisovalerate (due to deficiency of 3-MCC carboxylase); and propionate, 3-hydroxypropionate, methylcitrate, tiglylglycine (due to deficiency of PCC)	Severe metabolic acidosis, hyperammonemia, thrombocytopenia, seizures
HMG-CoA lyase deficiency	HMG-CoA lyase	HMG, 3-methylglutaconate, 3-hydroxyisovalerate, 3-methylglutarate	Severe metabolic acidosis without ketosis, hyperammonemia, hypoglycemia, macrocephaly
Glutaric aciduria, type II (multiple acyl-CoA dehydrogenase deficiency)	Electron transfer flavoprotein (ETF) or ETF dehydrogenase	Glutarate, ethylmalonate, methylsuccinate, isovalerylglycine, hexanoylglycine, butyrylglycine, isobutyrylglycine, 2-methylbutyryl glycine	Facial dysmorphism, cerebral dysgenesis, cystic kidneys

Table 8.3. (*cont.*)

3-Hydroxyisobutyric aciduria	3-Hydroxyisobutyryl-CoA dehydrogenase	3-Hydroxyisobutyrate, lactate	Facial dysmorphism, cerebral dysgenesis, hypotonia, failure to thrive, episodes of acidosis
5-Oxoprolinuria (Pyroglutamic aciduria)	Glutathione synthetase	5-Oxoproline (pyroglutamate)	Severe, persistent metabolic acidosis, hemolytic anemia, neutropenia
D-2-Hydroxyglutaric aciduria	D-2-Hydroxyglutaric acid transhydrogenase	D-2-Hydroxyglutaric acid	Seizures, infantile spasms (with hypsarrhythmia), chorioathetosis

Note: Abbreviations: HMG-CoA, 3-hydroxy-3-methylglutaryl-CoA; 3-MCC, 3-methylcrotonyl-CoA; PCC, propionyl-CoA carboxylase; PC, pyruvate carboxylase.

Infants with severe, neonatal-onset *holocarboxylase synthetase deficiency* present with many of the same clinical features as infants with propionic acidemia (Table 8.3), presumably because propionyl-CoA carboxylase is one of the enzymes affected by the defect in biotin metabolism. The urinary organic acid pattern, which shows high concentrations of the immediate precusors of each of the three catalytic carboxylases affected, is diagnostic of the disease. Treatment with pharmacologic doses of biotin reverses the metabolic abnormalities.

Infants with severe variants of *3-hydroxy-3-methylglutaryl-CoA (HMG-CoA) lyase deficiency* commonly present with rapidly progressing encephalopathy associated with severe metabolic acidosis, hypoketotic hypoglycemia, and hyperammonemia. Some biochemical evidence of hepatocellular dysfunction, with elevated bilirubin and transaminases, is also generally present. Urinary organic acid analysis shows large amounts of 3-hydroxy-3-methylglutarate, 3-methylglutaconate, 3-methylglutarate, and 3-hydroxyisovalerate. Diagnosis is confirmed by analysis of enzyme activity in cultured skin fibroblasts.

Severe encephalopathy, metabolic acidosis, hyperammonemia, along with facial dysmorphism, cerebral dysgenesis, and other anomalies, are features of severe *multiple acyl-CoA dehydrogenase deficiency* (glutaric aciduria, type II or GA II) and *3-hydroxyisobutyric aciduria* (see Chapter 7). Congenital visceral anomalies, such as renal cystic dysplasia, and hypoglycemia are characteristic of GA II and severe neonatal CPT II deficiency. All are rare conditions, particularly 3-hydroxyisobutyric aciduria. And all are generally rapidly fatal when they present in the newborn period. The diagnosis in each case is suggested by the results of urinary organic acid analysis and is confirmed by specific enzyme analysis in cultured skin fibroblasts.

Congenital lactic acidosis

The differentiation between the encephalopathy associated with congenital lactic acidosis, resulting either from primary defects of pyruvate metabolism or mitochondrial electron transport defects, and hypoxic-ischemic encephalopathy (HIE) may be difficult. Intractible seizures are commonly prominent in both. However, the clinical abnormalities and degree and duration of the lactic acidosis in newborns with defects in mitochondrial energy metabolism are usually out of proportion to the apparent severity of any hypoxic-ischemic insult experienced by the infant.

Signs that are particularly suggestive of severe primary congenital lactic acidosis include:

- small size for gestational age (SGA);
- subtle facial dysmorphism;

- structural malformations of the brain;
- multisystem disease (brain, kidney, liver, heart, eyes).

Simultaneous measurement of plasma lactate and pyruvate levels and calculation of the lactate/pyruvate (L/P) ratio is useful to distinguish pyruvate dehydrogenase (PDH) deficiency, in which the ratio is normal (15–20), from the severe neonatal form of pyruvate carboxylase deficiency (type B) and mitochondrial electron transport defects, in which the ratio is invariably >25. The L/P ratio is also normal in inborn errors of gluconeogenesis, such as glycogen storage disease, type I (GSD I) and *fructose-1,6-diphosphatase* (FDP) *deficiency,* which may sometimes present in the newborn period. However, they are associated with prominent hepatomegaly, hypoglycemia, and ketosis (in FDP deficiency), and encephalopathy is not present unless it is the result of severe, uncontrolled hypoglycemia (see section 'Hypoglycemia').

Many infants with severe *PDH deficiency* have facial dysmorphism suggestive of fetal alcohol syndrome: narrow skull with high bossed forehead, broad nasal bridge, small nose with anteverted nares, and large ears. In many cases, imaging studies of the brain show cerebral and cerebellar atrophy and cystic changes in the cerebrum and basal ganglia, and often agenesis or partial agenesis of the corpus callosum. The lactic acidosis in infants with PDH deficiency is often aggravated by high glucose intakes and ameliorated to some extent by high fat intakes. The diagnosis is confirmed by measurement of enzyme activity in leukocytes or cultured fibroblasts.

Unlike in older infants presenting with milder variants of pyruvate carboxylase deficiency (see Chapter 4), the L/P ratio in neonates with *pyruvate carboxylase, type B,* is elevated (>25). Postprandial ketoacidosis is a feature of this disorder, but the ratio of 3-hydroxybutyrate to acetoacetate is paradoxically decreased. Other prominent features are hyperammonemia and elevations of the plasma concentrations of the amino acids, citrulline, lysine, and proline, in addition to hyperalaninemia. The diagnosis is confirmed by enzyme assay in leukocytes or cultured skin fibroblasts.

Multisystem disease involvement is very suggestive of mitochondrial electron transport chain (ETC) defects, most commonly mitochondrial ETC complex I or complex IV (cytochrome *c* oxidase). One or more of skeletal myopathy, hypertrophic cardiomyopathy, hepatocellular dysfunction, renal tubular dysfunction, or cataracts are characteristic features of the neonatal variants of this class of diseases. The L/P ratio in these disorders is always elevated (>25). Imaging studies show that the brain is small with spongiform degenerative changes in the cerebrum and attenuation of white matter. Muscle biopsy in infants presenting this early does not show the ragged red fibers that are so typical of mitochondrial ETC defects presenting later in life. The diagnosis requires specialized studies on cultured fibroblasts or muscle (see Chapter 9). Most neonatal variants of the mitochondrial ETC defects are invariably and rapidly fatal. However, in a few patients, cytochrome c oxidase (complex IV) deficiency causing severe congenital lactic acidosis reverses spontaneously without serious permanent neurologic deficits.

Dicarboxylic aciduria

Pathologic dicarboxylic aciduria occurs most often as a manifestation of disorders of fatty acid oxidation (see Chapter 5). The clinical features of neonates presenting with fatty acid oxidation defects may be dominated by signs of any combination of encephalopathy, hepatocellular dysfunction, skeletal myopathy, or cardiomyopathy. Clinical generalizations about this group of inborn errors of metabolism must be regarded as provisional because the numbers of cases, particularly of patients presenting in the first few days or weeks of life, are very small. However, marked hypotonia and lethargy seem to be a feature of them all, and hepatomegaly is often prominent. Hypoketotic hypoglycemia, another characteristic feature of this class of disorders presenting in older infants, is common in affected neonates, and it is often accompanied by lactic acidosis, though this is not usually severe. Mild to moderately severe hyperammonemia is common. Plasma carnitine levels are decreased, and the esterified fraction is increased markedly. The urinary organic acid abnormalities, summarized in Table 8.3, are usually characteristic of the diseases.

Medium-chain acyl-CoA dehydrogenase (MCAD) deficiency, the commonest of the hereditary fatty acid oxidation defects in older infants (Chapter 5), is a very rare cause of severe illness in the newborn. It may be heralded by little more than marked hypotonia and mild lactic acidosis and hyperammonemia, without hypoglycemia or significant hepatomegaly. Urinary organic acid analysis shows the presence of large amounts of the medium-chain dicarboxylic acids (adipate, suberate, and sebacate) with very low levels of 3-hydroxybutyrate. Short-chain acyl-CoA dehydrogenase (SCAD) deficiency is characterized by nonspecific encephalopathy with poor feeding, failure to thrive, hypotonia, episodes of hypertonia and seizure-like activity, progressive muscle weakness and cardiomyopathy. Urinary organic acid analysis shows large amounts of ethyl-malonic acid, methylsuccinate, glutarate, butyrylglycine, and hexanoylglycine. The organic acid pattern is similar to that found in infants with GA II, or with cytochrome c oxidase deficiency.

Long-chain acyl-CoA dehydrogenase (LCAD) deficiency and long-chain hydroxyacyl-CoA dehydrogenase (LCHAD) deficiency, presenting in the new-born period, show encephalopathy, hepatocellular dysfunction, metabolic acidosis, hypoketotic hypoglycemia, and marked hypotonia. However, the prominence and severity of the cardiomyopathy, particularly in infants with LCHAD deficiency, sets this group apart from MCAD and SCAD deficiency. Urinary organic acid analysis shows large amounts of long-chain dicarboxylic and monocarboxylic acids in addition to medium-chain dicarboxylics. In the case of LCHAD deficiency, the 12-carbon and 14-carbon 3-hydroxydicarboxylic and monocarboxylic acids are particularly characteristic, though small amounts may sometimes be seen in infants with neonatal hepatitis.

Neonatal hepatic syndrome

The pattern of clinical abnormalities in patients with inherited metabolic disorders presenting with acute liver disease in the newborn period may be dominated by:

- jaundice;
- severe hepatocellular dysfunction (jaundice, hypoglycemia, hyperam-monemia, elevated transaminases, ascites and anasarca, and coagulopathy);
- hypoglycemia with little evidence of generalized hepatocellular dysfunction.

Jaundice

Jaundice is the principal, if not the only, sign of inborn errors of bilirubin metabolism, such as Gilbert syndrome, Lucey-Driscoll syndrome, Crigler-Najjar syndrome, and Dubin-Johnson syndrome (see Chapter 5). All are benign except for the type I variant of Crigler-Najjar syndrome, caused by total deficiency of hepatic uridine diphosphate (UDP)-glucuronosyltransferase. In-fants with this defect develop severe intractible unconjugated hyper-bilirubinemia within 24–48 hours of birth and invariably develop kernicterus.

In all other inherited metabolic conditions in which neonatal jaundice may be prominent, the hyperbilirubinemia is generally conjugated and is associated with other evidence of generalized hepatocellular dysfunction. Infants with *classical galactosemia* commonly present with a history of persistent hyperbilirubinemia. The hyperbilirubinemia is often unconjugated in the early stages of the disease, later becoming predominantly conjugated. The liver is enlarged and firm, and some evidence of hepatocellular dysfunction, sometimes severe, is invariably present, including hypoglycemia, elevated transaminases, mild to moderate coagulopathy, and mild hypoalbuminemia. Ascites is often seen, even in the absence of portal hypertension or hypoalbuminemia. Hyperchloremic metabolic acidosis, hypophosphatemia, and generalized amino aciduria indicate the presence of some renal tubular damage. Slit-lamp examination of the eyes often shows the presence of punctate lens opacities, even very early in the disease. These early cataracts generally resolve on treatment. Some infants with galactosemia present with severe cerebral edema and signs of intracranial hypertension. For reasons that are not well understood, infants with galactosemia are particularly susceptible to fulminant *Escherichia coli* sepsis. In fact, any infant with *E. coli* sepsis should be considered possibly to have the disease and be investigated accordingly.

The presence of nonglucose reducing substances in the urine in an infant with these findings is strong presumptive evidence of classical galactosemia. The galactosuria in infants with galactosemia is evanescent: if the infant has been off galactose-containing formula for more than a few hours, tests for nonglucose reducing substances are likely to be normal. Testing for reducing substances, using Clinitest tablets (Ames), can and should be done at the bedside at the earliest opportunity. Most hospitals caring for sick infants make available a galactosemia screening test, a semi-quantitative measurement of galactose-1-phosphate uridyltransferase (GALT) in red blood cells. Blood must be taken for this test before the infant receives any blood transfusions. Confirmation of the diagnosis is by quantitative analysis of GALT in red cells.

Galactosemia due to *generalized deficiency of UDPgalactose 4-epimerase* is extremely rare and clinically indistinguishable from classical galactosemia. In patients with 4-epimerase deficiency, galactosemia screening tests based on analysis of red cell galactose-1-phosphate may be positive, while those based on measurement of GALT activity are negative. The diagnosis is suggested by strong clinical evidence for galactosemia, including galactosuria, with normal GALT activity, and it is confirmed by measurement of 4-epimerase activity in cultured skin fibroblasts.

Infants with *alpha-1-antitrypsin deficiency* may present with persistent neonatal jaundice, predominantly conjugated and accompanied by other evidence of cholestasis. The jaundice commonly resolves spontaneously over a period of 6–10 weeks, and affected children often remain well until some months later when they present with evidence of cirrhosis with portal hypertension (see Chapter 5). The diagnosis may be suspected on the basis of the presence of typical inclusions in liver obtained by biopsy. Confirmation is based on demonstration of the presence of homozygosity for the protease inhibitor PI type ZZ phenotype.

Table 8.4. *Inherited metabolic diseases presenting with severe hepatocellular dysfunction in the newborn period.*

Disease	Associated findings	Distinguishing features
Amino acidopathies		
Hepatorenal tyrosinemia	Renal tubular dysfunction	Massive elevation of plasma α-fetoprotein; presence of succinylacetone in urine
Disorders of carbohydrate metabolism		
Hereditary fructose intolerance	Renal tubular dysfunction; lactic acidosis; hyperuricemia; hypoglycemia	History of exposure to fructose in the diet; deficiency of fructose-1-phosphate aldolase in liver
Glycogen storage disease, type IV	Hypoglycemia; severe coagulopathy	Severe generalized hepatocellular dysfunction; deficiency of hepatic glycogen brancher enzyme activity
Fatty acid oxidation defects		
MCAD deficiency	Hypoketotic hypoglycemia; encephalopathy	Medium-chain dicarboxylic aciduria
LCAD deficiency	Hypoketotic hypoglycemia; cardiomyopathy; encephalopathy	Long-chain monocarboxylic aciduria
LCHAD deficiency	Encephalopathy; cardiomyopathy	Long-chain 3-hydroxymono- and dicarboxylic aciduria
CPT II deficiency	Hypoketotic hypoglycemia; cardiomyopathy; encephalopathy; dysmorphic features; cystic kidneys; cardiac arrhythmias	Deficiency of CPT II in cultured fibroblasts
Carnitine-acylcarnitine translocase deficiency	Encephalopathy; metabolic acidosis; myopathy; cardiac arrhythmias	Marked elevation of plasma and urine long-chain acylcarnitines
Disorders of mitochondrial energy metabolism		
Cytochrome *c* oxidase deficiency	Encephalopathy; myopathy; lactic acidosis; retinitis pigmentosa; sensorineural hearing loss	Paradoxical increase in plasma ketones after meals; deficiency of cytochrome *c* oxidase in liver
Mitochondrial depletion syndrome	Myopathy; lactic acidosis; ketosis; renal tubular dysfunction	Marked depletion of mtDNA in muscle, brain, ±liver
Lysosomal storage diseases		
Niemann-Pick disease	Neonatal hepatitis	Storage histiocytes in bone marrow; deficiency of acid sphingomyelinase in type A and B variants; deficiency of cholesterol esterification in type C

Note: Abbreviations: MCAD, medium-chain acyl-CoA dehydrogenase; LCAD, long-chain acyl-CoA dehydrogenase; LCHAD, long-chain 3-hydroxyacyl-CoA dehydrogenase.

Severe hepatocellular dysfunction

Severe hepatocellular dysfunction due to inborn errors of metabolism presenting in early infancy is characterized by hypoglycemia, ascites, anasarca, hypoalbuminemia, hyperammonemia, hyperbilirubinemia (often only mild), and coagulopathy. The manifestations of liver disease are relatively nonspecific. Identification of the underlying defect is often based on recognition of specific secondary metabolic abnormalities (Table 8.4).

Hepatorenal tyrosinemia (hereditary tyrosinemia, type I), due to deficiency of fumarylacetoacetase (FAH), may present in the newborn period, though it more commonly presents later in infancy (Chapter 5). Presentation in the first few weeks of life is characterized by evidence of massive, acute hepatocellular dysfunction, along with evidence of renal tubular dysfunction (hyperchloremic metabolic acidosis, hypophosphatemia, glucosuria, and generalized amino aciduria). The liver is markedly enlarged, hard, and irregular in shape, a reflection of the degree of fibrosis already present at birth. Cardiomyopathy, sometimes severe enough to cause congestive heart failure, is common in infants with hepatorenal tyrosinemia.

Analysis of plasma amino acids shows increased levels of tyrosine, phenylalanine, and methionine, though the levels may not be significantly higher than in infants with other types of severe hepatocellular disease. Other biochemical abnormalities which support the diagnosis include depressed plasma cysteine levels and marked elevation of plasma α-fetoprotein levels. The coagulopathy of hepatorenal tyrosinemia is characterized by dysfibrinogenemia which is reflected in dysproportionate prolongation of the reptilase time compared with the thrombin time. Urinary organic acid analysis usually shows the presence of succinylacetone, which is a specific characteristic of the disease. The absence of succinylacetone in the urine does not exclude the diagnosis of hepatorenal tyrosinemia. If the clinical suspicion is high, urinary organic acid analysis should be repeated at least several times and fumarylacetoacetase activity should be measured in leukocytes or fresh liver tissue.

The association of encephalopathy with evidence of moderately severe hepatocellular dysfunction and cardiomyopathy are features of *fatty acid oxidation defects* (FAOD) which may make them difficult to distinguish from hepatorenal tyrosinemia. Generalized hypotonia, the result of the involvement of skeletal muscle, may be profound in both. However, biosynthetic defects (hypoalbumin and coaguloapthy) are not as prominent in infants with hepatopathy due to fatty acid oxidation defects, and the cardiomyopathy is generally much more severe, *except* in MCAD deficiency, sometimes progressing rapidly to intractible congestive heart failure, cardiac arrythmias, and death.

Plasma α-fetoprotein levels are not elevated, and renal tubular function is not disturbed. Urinary organic acid analysis shows the presence of aromatic tyrosine metabolites and fatty acid oxidation intermediates, similar to those seen in older children with fatty acid oxidation defects (see Chapter 5), but succinylacetone is not found, regardless of the severity of the liver disease. The organic acid abnormalities in infants with fatty acid oxidation defects are notoriously evanescent. They may clear early, making the presumptive diagnosis on the basis of urinary organic acid analysis very difficult. In these situations, analysis of plasma acylcarnitines by high resolution, tandem MS–MS analysis is particularly helpful. The diagnosis and classification of the FAOD is generally confirmed by analysis of fatty acid oxidation in cultured skin fibroblasts (see Chapter 9).

The clinical features of acute, neonatal hepatorenal tyrosinemia and early-onset variants of the hereditary fatty acid oxidation defects may be difficult to distinguish from *neonatal hemachromatosis* or *neonatal hepatitis*. In both these acquired conditions, plasma α-fetoprotein levels may be very high, though not usually as high as in tyrosinemia. Urinary organic acid analysis will show the presence of the same mixture of aromatic tyrosine metabolites that occurs in tyrosinemia as a result of severe hepatocellular dysfunction, but the presence of succinylacetone is specific for hepatorenal tyrosinemia. The histopathologic appearances of tissue obtained by liver biopsy are also different in the three diseases.

The association of acute hepatocellular dysfunction (hypoglycemia, hepatomegaly, elevated transaminases), severe lactic acidosis, hyperuricemia, hypophosphatemia, and hyperchloremic metabolic acidosis with the ingestion of fructose is characteristic of hereditary fructose intolerance (HFI) presenting in the newborn period. The hypoglycemia and lactic acidosis may be severe enough to be life-threatening. Presentation of HFI in the newborn period has become much less common now that neonates requiring supplementation are given oral glucose solution rather than sugar-water containing sucrose. Enzymic confirmation of the diagnosis is difficult because the deficient enzyme (fructose-1-phosphate aldolase) is confined to liver. Fructose loading tests are dangerous and should not be done.

Defects in the acylcarnitine synthesis-translocation-hydrolysis process (Chapter 5), such as carnitine palmitoyltransferase I (CPT I) deficiency, CPT II deficiency, or carnitine-acylcarnitine translocase deficiency, generally present with severe hepatomegaly and hepatocellular dysfunction, along with encephalopathy, hyperammonemia, hypoketotic hypoglycemia, metabolic acidosis, and hypotonia. Cardiac arrhythmias appear to be a prominent feature of translocase deficiency. Unlike the other inherited defects of fatty acid oxidation, the urinary organic acids are usually completely normal, and the plasma carnitine concentration is usually *elevated*. In CPT I deficiency, the acylcarnitines are not remarkable; however, in translocase deficiency, the concentration of long-chain acylcarnitines in plasma is grossly elevated. Mitochondrial depletion syndrome may present with similar clinical findings. However, affected infants are usually severely ketotic.

We have managed two infants presenting with severe cirrhosis in the first week of life because of glycogen storage disease, type IV (GSD IV). The total failure of biosynthetic functions was particularly remarkable. Disease presenting this early is invariably rapidly fatal, and diagnosis is generally confirmed by the typical histopathologic findings in the liver and biochemical studies done at autopsy.

Many infants who present later in infancy or early childhood with neurologic or hepatic abnormalities of Niemann-Pick disease, irrespective of the variant of the disease, have a history of persistent neonatal jaundice. The histopathologic changes in liver obtained by biopsy are often indistinguishable from giant cell hepatitis. The jaundice and associated hepatomegaly generally resolve spontaneously over a period of several days or a few weeks.

Hypoglycemia

Hypoglycemia is a frequent, nonspecific complication of almost any severe illness in the newborn. Prematurity, intrauterine growth retardation, maternal diabetes mellitus, sepsis, and asphyxia are just a few of the common conditions associated with symptomatic hypoglycemia. The underlying disorder is generally obvious and the blood glucose is relatively easy to control. Hypoglycemia may also be prominent, though generally not difficult to control, in infants with adrenal insufficiency or growth hormone deficiency. The hypoglycemia occurring as a result of hyperinsulinism caused by nesidioblastosis is typically much more difficult to correct, requiring iv glucose infusion rates exceeding 12 mg/kg body weight/minute, or administration of glucagon, to control. Infusion of glucose at rates exceeding 12 mg/kg/minute often produces lactic acidosis, which may cause diagnostic confusion unless the relationship with the rapid infusion of glucose is noted.

In many of the inherited metabolic diseases that may be associated with neonatal hypoglycemia, instability of the blood glucose is a relatively trivial matter compared with other problems, like metabolic acidosis and hyperammonemia or severe hepatocellular dysfunction. However, hypoglycemia is often the only sign of disease in infants with primary disorders of gluconeogenesis presenting in the first week or two of life. The hypoglycemia is clearly related to fasting, and, although it may be severe, it is typically relatively easy to control with nothing more than regular feeds at intervals of three to four hours.

GSD I may present in the newborn period with hypoglycemia associated with lactic acidosis. The hypoglycemia is usually easy to control by intravenous administration of relatively small amounts of glucose (<6–7 mg/kg/min), or frequent feeds. As soon as an infant with GSD I is able to tolerate full feeds, symptomatic hypoglycemia generally resolves only to reappear at three to four months of age when attempts are made to extend the interval between feeds. The liver of infants with the disease may be normal or only slightly enlarged during the first few days of life. However, by one week of age, often after the hypoglycemia occurring in the first few days of life has been controlled, the liver becomes markedly enlarged. The diagnosis is suggested by the association of hypoglycemia with lactic acidosis and hyperuricemia. In GSD, type Ib, the neutropenia characteristic of the disease develops within the first few days of life, though increased susceptibility to infection may not become a problem until some months later. The diagnosis of GSD I is supported by failure of the hypoglycemia to respond to injections of glucagon. Confirmation requires liver biopsy and measurement of glucose-6-phosphatase in fresh tissue or hitochemically, bearing in mind that special studies are necessary to make the diagnosis of GSD Ib and Ic (see Chapter 5).

Hypoglycemia resulting from other defects in gluconeogenesis, such as fructose-1,6-diphosphatase (FDP) deficiency, is less common, but may be clinically indistinguishable from GSD, type Ia. Massive hepatomegaly, marked intolerance of fasting, lactic acidosis, hyperuricemia, and ketotis are features of both; however, ketosis is generally much more prominent in FDP deficiency.

Nonimmune fetal hydrops

The list of conditions associated with nonimmune fetal hydrops is long and includes a number of genetic disorders, in addition to severe anemia, congenital heart disease, and congenital infection. In a significant proportion of cases, an underlying explanation for it is never found. A small proportion of the total are the result of inherited metabolic diseases (Table 8.5). The hydrops associated with inborn errors of red blood cell energy metabolism is undoubtedly the result of heart failure precipitated by severe anemia. The relationship between fluid accumulation, heart failure, and anemia is obvious, and investigation of the hematologic disorder generally identifies the underlying defect.

The birth weight of infants with lysosomal storage diseases, particularly the mucopolysaccharidoses, is sometimes excessive and associated with some noticeable swelling of the extremities. Marked weight loss often occurs during the first several days of life as accumulated subcutaneous fluid is resorbed and excreted. Why some newborn infants with lysosomal storage diseases are born with massive generalized edema and ascites is not clear. Severely affected infants

Table 8.5. *Inherited metabolic diseases presenting as nonimmune fetal hydrops.*

Hematologic disorders
G6PD deficiency
Pyruvate kinase deficiency
Glucosephosphate isomerase deficiency

Lysosomal storage diseases
GM1 gangliosidosis
Gaucher disease
Niemann-Pick disease
Sialidosis
Galactosialidosis
I-cell disease
Sialic acid storage disorder
Morquio disease (MPS IV)
Sly disease (MPS VII)

Note: Abbreviations: G6PD, glucose-6-phosphate dehydrogenase.

usually go on to die as a result of respiratory embarrassment, circulatory failure, or coagulopathies. In a few milder cases, the fluid accumulation resolves spontaneously. The presence of dysostosis multiplex, marked hepatosplenomegaly, vacuolated mononuclear cells in the peripheral smear, and storage histiocytes in bone marrow or other tissues are strongly suggestive of a lysosomal storage disease. However, definitive diagnosis invariably requires enzyme analyses of cultured skin fibroblasts or tissues.

Initial management
Early and aggressive management of many inherited metabolic diseases is often life-saving. The principles of initial management are summarized in Table 8.6.

Eliminate dietary or other intake of the precursors of possibly toxic metabolites. This applies most often to suspected inborn errors of amino acid or organic acid metabolism. In both cases, dietary or parenteral intake of protein and amino acids should be eliminated immediately an inborn error of metabolism is suspected. Because inherited disorders of fatty acid oxidation may not initially be easily distinguished from the amino acidopathies, dietary and intravenous fat intake should also be eliminated, at least initially.

*Administer a metabolically simple source of **calories**, i.e. glucose, at a rate sufficient to suppress mobilization of endogenous sources of the metabolites, especially protein.* In acute, metabolically decompensated MSUD, the goal should be to provide 100 cal/kg/day intravenously. This is achieved by the intravenous

Table 8.6. *Initial management of possible inherited metabolic diseases presenting in the newborn period.*

Principle	Specific initiative
Minimize intake and endogenous production of toxic metabolites	Eliminate protein and fat from the diet Administer high calorie, high carbohydrate intravenous fluids: 10% dextrose in 0.2% NaCl at 1.5 times calculated maintenance, and add KCl when urinary output is established
Correct acidosis	Administer intravenous sodium bicarbonate CAUTIOUSLY if plasma bicarbonate is <10 mmol/L
Treat intercurrent illness	
In the presence of intractible seizures without hyperammonemia or metabolic acidosis	Pyridoxine, 100–200 mg iv
Accelerate elimination of toxic metabolites	Hemodialysis Continuous venous-venous hemoperfusion
In the presence of suspected urea cycle enzyme defect	Administer arginine hydrochloride, 2–4 mmoles/kg, iv over one hour followed by 2–4 mmol/kg/24 hours in 4 divided doses* Administer sodium benzoate, 250 mg/kg, iv immediately followed by 250 mg/kg/24 hours in 4 divided doses† Administer sodium phenylacetate, 250 mg/kg, iv immediately followed by 250 mg/kg/24 hours in 4 divided doses†

Note: * Arginine hydrochloride, which is generally readily available in most hospital pharmacies, should be replaced by arginine-free base as soon as possible to avoid hydrochloride-induced metabolic acidosis.
† Sodium benzoate and sodium phenylacetate are available as a pre-mixed preparation called Ucephan.

administration of 10% dextrose supplemented by Intralipid. Intravenous lipid is specifically contraindicated in children with suspected defects in fatty acid oxidation, although some of these patients may turn out to have defects (such as systemic carnitine deficiency) responsive to replacement of usual dietary fat by medium chain triglyceride (MCT) oil.

*Administer greater than maintenance amounts of **fluids** to promote diuresis and* *accelerate excretion of water-soluble, toxic metabolites.* Care must be taken to avoid fluid over-load in children with acute, encephalopathic MSUD or UCED.

Treat shock, hypoglycemia, metabolic acidosis, electrolyte imbalances, infections, and coagulopathies by conventional methods. Metabolic acidosis should be treated cautiously. Bicarbonate is generally not indicated unless the plasma bicarbonate is <10 mmol/L; deficits should be only half corrected.

In cases involving potentially vitamin responsive enzymopathies, administer pharmacologic doses of the relevant vitamin. This is most important in the treatment of suspected pyridoxine dependency seizures of the newborn. As a general rule, vitamin responsive enzymopathies are clinically less severe than nonresponsive variants. A trial of therapy with vitamins would be indicated nevertheless in any acutely ill patient in whom a strong presumptive diagnosis of a specific, potentially vitamin-responsive, inborn error of metabolism is made.

Administer pharmacologic agents known to detoxify or accelerate the excretion of toxic metabolites. The efficacy of nontoxic drugs, such as sodium benzoate and sodium phenylacetate, that accelerate nitrogen excretion in patients with UCED by forming innocuous, rapidly-cleared amino acid conjugates (hippuric acid and phenylacetylglutamine, respectively) is well established.

Consider dialysis for treatment of resistant, life-threatening metabolic acidosis, rapidly progressive encephalopathy, or treatment-induced electrolyte disturbances, e.g., hypernatremia. Patients with UCED presenting in the newborn period with severe hyperammonemia usually require hemodialysis or CVVH to control ammonium levels. Peritoneal dialysis is too slow. Exchange transfusion brings the plasma ammonium down quickly, but rebound hyperammonemia occurs just as quickly. It may be useful in some circumstances as an adjunct to dialysis.

Summary comments

Treatable inherited metabolic diseases often present in early infancy or childhood as acute, life-threatening illness. Diagnosis is often delayed, however, because the conditions are individually rare, the presenting signs and symptoms are often nonspecific, and diagnosis usually rests on biochemical testing that may not be readily available. This chapter presents an approach to the problem that stresses those clinical signs or situations which should suggest the strong possibility of disease due to inborn errors of metabolism, the initial investigation of infants or children suspected of being affected with an inherited metabolic disease, and the initial management of the patient. The approach is based on experience that suggests diagnosis is often unnecessarily delayed because premonitory signs are misinterpreted, that a clinically useful presumptive diagnosis can often be made with the aid of relatively easily accessible laboratory facilities, and that effective initial managment of affected infants and children, while relatively nonspecific, allows time for more definitive investigation and specific, long-term treatment.

Bibliography

Brusilow, S.W., Batshaw, M.L. & Waber, L. (1982). Neonatal hyperammonemic coma. *Advances in Pediatrics*, **29**, 69–102.

Burton, B.K. (1987). Inborn errors of metabolism: the clinical diagnosis in early infancy. *Pediatrics*, **79**, 359–69.

Clayton, P.T. & Thompson, E. (1988). Dysmorphic syndromes with demonstrable biochemical abnormalities. *Journal of Medical Genetics*, **25**, 463–72.

Goodman, S.I. (1986). Inherited metabolic disease in the newborn: approach to diagnosis and treatment. *Advances in Pediatrics*, **33**, 197–224.

Hudak, M.L., Jones, Jr., M.D. & Brusilow, S.W. (1985). Differentiation of transient hyperammonemia of the newborn and urea cycle enzyme defects by clinical presentation. *Journal of Pediatrics*, **107**, 712–19.

Kurnetz, R., Yang, S., Holmes, R. & Harrison, D.D. (1985). Neonatal jaundice and coagulopathy. *Journal of Pediatrics*, **107**, 982–7.

Leonard, J.V. (1985). The early detection and management of inborn errors presenting acutely in the neonatal period. *European Journal of Pediatrics*, **143**, 253–7.

Robinson, B.H., MacMillan, H., Petrova-Benedict, R. & Sherwood, W.G. (1987). Variable clinical presentation in patients with defective E1 component of pyruvate dehydrogenase complex. *Journal of Pediatrics*, **111**, 525–33.

Saudubray, J.M., Narcy, C., Lyonnet, L., Bonnefont, J.P., Poll-The, B.T. & Munnich, A. (1990). Clinical approach to inherited metabolic disorders in neonates. *Biology of the Neonate*, **58(suppl. 1)**, 44–53.

Saudubray, J.M. & Charpentier, C. (1995). Clinical phenotypes: diagnosis/algorithms. In *The Metabolic and Molecular Bases of Inherited Disease*, 7th edn, ed. C.R. Scriver, A.L. Beaudet, W.S. Sly & D. Valle, pp. 327–400. New York: McGraw-Hill, Inc.

Ward, J.C. (1990). Inborn errors of metabolism of acute onset in infancy. *Pediatrics in Review*, **11**, 205–16.

9

Laboratory investigation

It is impossible to exaggerate the importance of the diagnostic clinical chemisty laboratory in the investigation of inherited metabolic diseases. Access to comprehensive routine laboratory testing is indispensable to the establishment of the diagnosis of any suspected inherited metabolic condition, and the clinical biochemist is an extremely important collaborator whose allegiance should be cultivated carefully. In this chapter, I present information relating to the laboratory investigation of inherited metabolic diseases to help the clinician understand some of the technical principles involved, to give enough detail about certain tests to provide a feel for the interpretation of test results, and some of the more common sources of error. It is not intended to be a detailed technical treatise on clinical chemistry. However, I have found that the initial laboratory investigation of patients with possible inborn errors of metabolism is generally more appropriate when the clinician has some understanding of laboratory issues. Separating off some of the diagnostic laboratory information in a separate chapter like this does create its own problems. Specifically, it is difficult at times to decide whether a particular point should be included here, or if it would not be more logically placed alongside of the presentation of the clinical aspects of a particular disease. This has been resolved in most cases by a compromise. If the laboratory aspects, of for example amino acid analysis, are relevant to more than one major clinical presentation, such as chronic encephalopathy (covered in Chapter 2), hyperphenylalaninemia (Chapter 3), metabolic acidosis (Chapter 4), and hepatocellular dysfunction (Chapter 5), it seemed more appropriate to place it in a separate chapter. However, the physiologic rationale for some laboratory studies seemed more appropriate in the chapter in which presentation of the information would be helpful in grasping the pathophysiology of a particular disease.

Laboratory chemists supervise the technical aspects of specific testing. They not only provide information regarding the availability and appropriateness of specific tests, the limitations of the investigation, and the interpretation of the results, they can often influence the scheduling of testing so that results that are needed urgently are obtained with a minimum of delay. When certain specialized testing is not available locally, the clinical chemist is often the one who knows where it can be obtained and will facilitate referral to an appropriate reference laboratory.

The goal of various laboratory studies, including biochemical testing, may be to:

- determine the extent and severity of organ or tissue involvement;
- classify a presumed inherited metabolic problem according to the aspect of metabolism involved;
- establish a specific diagnosis.

The types of tests that might be undertaken to determine what organs or tissues are involved in a disease process, and the severity of the involvement, include the wide range of biochemical, hematologic, electrophysiologic, imaging, and histopathologic studies which are useful for the assessment of any disorder, inherited or acquired. They include routine biochemical tests like measurements of arterial blood gases, plasma electrolytes, glucose, urea, creatinine, liver function tests, routine hematologic tests, and various endocrinologic tests, such as thyroxine, triiodothyronine, thyroid stimulating hormone. They also include somewhat more specialized electrophysiologic studies, such as EEG, evoked potentials, EMG, and nerve conduction studies, as well as ECG. Imaging studies that are particularly helpful, though not specific to the investigation of inherited metabolic disorders, include routine skeletal radiography, echocardiography, CT scanning, and magnetic resonance imaging. Histopathologic, histochemical, and ultrastructural studies are particularly useful in the investigation of inherited disorders of organelle function and metabolism (see Chapter 7).

A number of somewhat less readily available biochemical tests are used to identify metabolic abnormalities and classify them according to the general area or pathway of metabolism involved. The tests are generally not specific enough to differentiate primary from secondary metabolic abnormalities, though the pattern of abnormalities may be suggestive of a specific diagnosis. Studies in this category include measurements of lactate, pyruvate, amino acids, 3-hydroxybutyrate, acetoacetate, and free fatty acids in plasma; analyses of urinary organic and amino acids; tests for mucopolysacchariduria and oligosacchariduria; and measurements of certain trace elements, such as copper.

The ultimate specific diagnosis of inherited metabolic disease generally requires the demonstration of a primary biochemical abnormality, such as a specific enzyme deficiency, or mutations that have been demonstrated to cause

Table 9.1. *Clinical differentiation of organelle disease and small molecule disease.*

Feature	Organelle disease	Small molecule disease
Onset	Gradual	Often sudden, even catastrophic
Course	Slowly progressive	Characterized by relapses and remissions
Physical findings	Characteristic features	Nonspecific
Histopathology	Often reveals characteristic changes	Generally nonspecific changes
Response to supportive therapy	Poor	Brisk

disease. These tests are generally available only in large metropolitan teaching hospitals or university medical centers.

A useful first step in helping to focus the laboratory investigation of possible inherited metabolic diseases is to try to determine whether the disease is due to a defect in the metabolism of water-soluble intermediates, such as amino acids, organic acids, or other low molecular weight compounds, or is likely due to an inherited defect of organelle metabolism, such as lysosomal, mitochondrial, or peroxisomal metabolism. Table 9.1 summarizes some features that are helpful in differentiating the two classes of disorders.

The *onset of signs of disease* is an important, though not infallible, clue to the nature of the underlying disorder. Diseases presenting with a sudden or catastrophic onset are generally more likely to be attributable to inherited defects of small molecule metabolism. Catastrophic deterioration on a background of chronic disease is also more likely to be due to small molecule disorders, particularly if the clinical history is one of recurrent exacerbations and remissions separated by periods of relatively good health. However, the interpretation of the diagnostic significance of sudden deterioration requires some care. The disease process in patients with organelle disease may erode the general health of the patient, or the function of some specific organ or tissue, to the extent that intercurrent infections or otherwise trivial illnesses cause generalized organelle dysfunction or severe organ failure. An example is acute deterioration of patients with mitochondrial disorders occurring as a result of sudden metabolic decompensation in the face of an otherwise trivial viral illness. An acute-on-chronic presentation is not, therefore, invariably an indication that the underlying defect is in small molecule metabolism.

Table 9.2. *Some general clinical characteristics of defects of organelle metabolism.*

Lysosomal	Peroxisomal	Mitochondrial
Disease limited to nervous system ± RES	Multisystem disease	Multisystem disease
Chronic course	Failure to thrive	Failure to thrive
Hepatosplenomegaly, variable	Profound hypotonia	Cerebral dysgenesis
Leukodystrophy, often severe	Cerebral dysgenesis	Sensorineural hearing loss
Cerebellar atrophy, marked	Hepatocellular dysfunction	Peripheral neuropathy
Skin lesions (angiokeratomata)	Sensorineural hearing loss	Myopathy
'Cherry red' macular spot	Neuropathy	Extraocular ophthalmoplegia
Behavior/psychiatric problems	Cystic disease of kidneys	Cardiomyopathy
Seizures, late	Seizures, early and intractible	Retinitis pigmentosa
		Seizures, variable

Note: Abbreviation: RES, reticuloendothelial system.

Similarly, although a gradual onset of symptoms is characteristic of many organelle disorders, like lysosomal storage diseases and peroxisomal disorders, it is also a feature of some of the small molecule diseases, especially some of the amino acidopathies, like phenylketonuria (PKU) and homocystinuria. In this case, the course of the disease must be considered in the light of other clinical findings, such as the presence or absence of what might be characterized as particular physical findings or dysmorphic features.

The presence of *specific physical findings or dysmorphic features* suggests in general that the underlying defect is in organelle metabolism. While the generalization may hold most of the time, there are also some important exceptions. Urinary organic acid analysis would usually be regarded as a 'small molecule' test. However, some of the inherited metabolic diseases associated with diagnostic organic aciduria, such as mevalonic aciduria and glutaric aciduria type II, often present with severe dysmorphism. Among the various inherited disorders of organelle metabolism, the type and extent of tissue and organ involvement often provides a clue to which organelle might be implicated (Table 9.2). Here again, the summary information presented in Table 9.2 is intended to serve only as a guide; there are many exceptions to these generalizations. For example, hypertrophic cardiomyopathy is a common manifestation of mitochondrial cytopathies. However, it is often the presenting sign of GSD II, a lysosomal storage disorder.

Specific histopathologic or ultrastructural abnormalities may be sufficiently characteristic to permit a strong presumptive diagnosis in many of the organelle diseases. Often microscopic examination of tissues or organs not obviously involved with the disease provides invaluable diagnostic information in these cases. For example, the clinical abnormalities in neuronal ceroid lipofuscinosis are confined to the central nervous system (CNS). However, electron microscopic examination of conjunctival mucosa, skin, peripheral blood lymphocytes, or rectal mucosa, generally shows the presence of the typical lysosomal inclusions that are diagnostic of the disease (see Figure 2.2). Bone marrow examination generally provides histopathologic information specific enough to make a strong presumptive diagnosis of Gaucher disease (see Figure 7.5) or Niemann-Pick disease. Histopathologic and ultrastructural abnormalities may be present in patients with small molecule disorders, but as a rule they are not sufficiently specific to provide a diagnosis.

The *response to aggressive supportive measures*, or 'first-aid', is also different between the organelle diseases and the small molecule disorders. The administration of intravenous fluids, glucose, maintenance electrolytes, and correction of metabolic acidosis, often results in significant early, if not dramatic, improvement of patients with small molecule disease who may be acutely ill as a result of metabolic decompensation. In contrast, patients with organelle disease generally respond slowly and incompletely to supportive measures unless deterioration is sudden and the cause is immediately obvious and correctable, such as acute airway obstruction.

Studies on the extent and severity of pathology
Studies directed at determining the extent and severity of organ or tissue failure are generally nonspecific, although the pattern or distribution of abnormalities may be suggestive of a specific disease. Most imaging studies, such as radiographs, MRI, CT scans, and ultrasound examinations, are in this category. Electrophysiologic studies are also relatively nonspecific, showing that a system is affected by disease, but not usually shedding much light on the basic defect. Routine biochemical studies are also generally nonspecific, though they are often helpful in classifying metabolic defects.

Studies directed at the classification of disease processes (the 'metabolic screen')

In the interests of simplifying the investigation of the possibility of inborn errors of metabolism, many laboratories and hospitals have developed customized batteries of screening tests which are grouped together as a 'metabolic screen'. What is included in the battery of tests varies from one laboratory to another, creating the potential for confusion. One of the main problems with so-called metabolic screens is the potentially false sense of security they may produce in the minds of physicians who may not appreciate the limitations of the screening battery. Metabolic screens are probably here to stay, and it is important to determine for each laboratory what tests are included in the test battery and how to interpret the results in each case.

Tests in this category include analysis of plasma ammonium, plasma lactate, pyruvate, 3-hydroxybutyrate, and free fatty acids, quantitative or semi-quantitative analysis of plasma and urine amino acids, urinary or plasma organic acid analysis, urinary mucopolysaccharide (MPS) and oligosaccharide screening tests, and galactosemia screening tests. Definitive diagnosis generally requires further *in vitro* metabolic studies, usually specific enzyme assay. The principles involved in the various analytic techniques are described here, along with some indications of interpretation of test results and major sources of error.

Investigation of 'small molecule disease'

Plasma ammonium

The measurement of plasma ammonium in most laboratories is now done enzymatically with the aid of an autoanalyzer, eliminating the delays and inherent inaccuracies associated with older spectrophotometric methods. However, the determination of plasma ammonium levels is still subject to significant errors arising from environmental contamination, poor venipuncture technique, and careless sample handling. Blood samples should be drawn from a free flowing vein directly into an anticoagulated tube, placed immediately on ice, and the plasma separated and analysis performed within 15 minutes of the blood being drawn. Normal plasma ammonium concentrations vary somewhat with age, being slightly higher in newborn infants.

Plasma lactate and pyruvate

Plasma lactate and pyruvate levels are generally analyzed enzymatically. The same precautions required for accurate measurement of plasma ammonium apply to measurements of plasma lactate. The use of a tourniquet and delayed sample handling are common causes of spurious elevations of plasma lactate.

Lactate levels in arterial blood and cerebrospinal fluid (CSF) are generally more reliable than venous plasma lactates. The measurement of pyruvate in plasma is cumbersome, and the results are seriously prone to error. Pyruvate levels in blood are always at least an order of magnitude lower than lactate levels, and pyruvate in blood is unstable. Lactate to pyruvate ratios in plasma should, therefore, be interpreted with care.

Plasma ketones and free fatty acids

Plasma ketones (3-hydroxybutyrate and acetoacetate) are measured enzymatically. 3-Hydroxybutyrate in plasma is relatively stable stored frozen at $-20°C$. However, acetoacetate is unstable, and quantitative analysis is technically more difficult than measurement of 3-hydroxybutyrate. Because of the technical difficulties associated with acetoacetate measurements, and the finding that pathologic increases in plasma ketone levels characteristically affect 3-hydroxybutyrate more than acetoacetate, many laboratories offer quantitative measurements only of the former. Semi-quantitative methods for estimating blood ketone levels, with the use of Acetest tablets or Ketostix (Ames), measure acetoacetate only; 3-hydroxybutyrate, the principal ketone in blood, does not react.

Free fatty acids in plasma can be measured in many ways. However, most manual methods are cumbersome and are being replaced by semi-automated assays based on colorimetric measurement of cupric ion binding. This method is not appropriate for the analysis of very long-chain fatty acids in the investigation of inherited defects of peroxisomal metabolism.

Amino acid analysis

The capability to detect amino acid abnormalities in various physiologic fluids, like plasma, urine and CSF, is central to the investigation of possible inherited metabolic diseases. The detection of abnormalities may be by:

- some relatively nonspecific chemical reactions producing colored reaction products;
- paper or thin-layer chromatography coupled with staining with ninhydrin and other reagents producing colored products upon reaction with specific amino acids;
- ion-exchange chromatography, the basis of most automated amino acid analyzers used for the amino acid quantitation of physiologic fluids;
- high performance liquid chromatography (HPLC), most useful in the analysis of cleaner samples, such as protein hydrolysates;

- gas chromatography-mass spectrometry (GC–MS);
- high resolution, tandem mass spectrometry-mass spectrometry (MS–MS).

Many metabolic screens include a selection of relatively nonspecific chemical tests for the presence of compounds containing certain functional groups. In some laboratories, these are combined with, or replaced by, thin-layer or paper chromatography of urine, plasma, or blood to screen for amino acid abnormalities in low-risk patients or as an adjunct to quantitative amino acid analysis, usually by ion-exchange chromatography. HPLC analysis of amino acids in protein hydrolysates is rapid, accurate, and relatively inexpensive. However, the presence of large amounts of interfering substances makes application of the method to the analysis of free amino acids in physiologic fluids less reliable. Most clinical laboratories doing amino acid quantitation still use ion-exchange chromatography as the principal analytic methodology.

High resolution tandem MS–MS is rapid, accurate, and requires only small samples of blood. A significant advantage of mass spectrometry is the wide range of chemically unrelated compounds and metabolites which can be analyzed simultaneously in extremely small samples of the relevant physiologic fluid, such as dried blood spots. The potential capacity of this methodology, coupled with low operating costs and rapid turnaround times, makes this a potentially powerful tool for centralized state screening laboratories.

Chemical screening tests for aminoaciduria

A number of tests have evolved for rapid detection of specific classes of amino acids or amino acid metabolites (Table 9.3). They are inexpensive, require only small amounts of urine, and are technically simple to perform. They are even adaptable for use at home, in certain circumstances, for monitoring therapy. In general, they are relatively insensitive and nonspecific, being affected by the presence of a wide range of compounds, such as drug metabolites. They provide useful initial screening tests, but the results must be interpreted with care.

Paper or thin-layer chromatography

Paper or thin-layer chromatographic separation of amino acids in blood, plasma, or urine, and visualization by treatment with ninhydrin is an excellent technique for detecting *excesses* of single amino acids, such as phenylalanine or tyrosine, or small groups of structurally related amino acids, such as the branched-chain amino acids. It is next to useless for the detection of *deficiencies* of amino acids, a feature that seriously compromises the usefulness of this type of analysis in the investigation of possible urea cycle enzyme defects. Artifacts are common, but generally they are readily recognizable.

Staining with ninhydrin is generally carried out to visualize all the amino acids. Accurate interpretation of the chromatogram requires appreciation of possible presence of various confounding amino acid-like compounds. Additional stains are used to detect specific amino acids (Table 9.4).

Quantitative amino acid analysis

Quantitative amino acid analysis by semi-automated ion-exchange chromatography with the use of any of the commercially available instruments specifically designed for analysis of physiologic fluids is an indispensable component of any diagnostic service involved with the management of inherited metabolic diseases. It meets four important needs:

- It provides for the confirmation of the identity and concentration of abnormal ninhydrin-positive compounds that might have been detected by any of the screening tests discussed above.
- When it is readily accessible, it ends up to be faster than paper or thin-layer chromatographic analysis.
- It provides accurate quantitative information on the levels of amino acids which may be present in *subnormal* concentrations, in addition to those that are present in excess.
- It is the only way of quantitating reliably the concentrations of amino acids in physiologic fluids, like CSF, in which the levels of all amino acids are normally very low.

Secondary abnormalities of amino acid concentrations in plasma and urine are very common. Severe hepatocellular disease, renal tubular disease, catabolic states, pregnancy, vitamin deficiencies, malnutrition, neoplasia, infection, burns, and injuries are all associated with disturbances of amino acid concentrations in plasma or urine or both. Sorting out whether a particular abnormality is due to an inborn error of metabolism or secondary to some commonly acquired disorder is sometimes difficult. In many cases, the matter is resolvable by eliciting a history of injury, stress, or disease. However, in some, the distinction between abnormalities attributable to primary metabolic disease and secondary metabolic responses to acquired disease requires further investigation. This is especially true when a particular inherited disorder of amino acid metabolism, such as hepatorenal tyrosinemia, causes severe generalized or organ-specific tissue damage. In other instances, primary inherited disorders of fat, organic acid, or carbohydrate metabolism are associated with secondary disturbances of amino

Table 9.3. *Chemical screening tests for amino acids and amino acid metabolites in urine.*

Screening test	Compound	Interpretation
Ferric chloride or Phenistix	Phenylpyruvic acid	Typical stable green color occurs in untreated PKU. Other conditions or the presence of a wide range of interfering metabolites (e.g., p-hydroxyphenylpyruvic acid, branched chain ketoacids, imidazolepyruvic acid, homogentisic acid) or drugs (e.g., acetaminophen, salicylates, phenothiazines, isoniazid) produce different colors
Dinitrophenylhydrazine	α-Ketoacids	Typical yellow precipitate occurs in MSUD, PKU, or ketoacidosis
Cyanide nitroprusside	Disulfide bonds	Rapid development of red-purple color occurs in cystinuria, homocystinuria, or β-mercaptolactate-cysteine disulfiduria. The ingestion of certain drugs, notably N-acetylcysteine (Mucomyst), penicillamine, captopril, or synthetic penicillins, also produces a positive reaction. Atypical color reactions occur in ketoacidosis
Nitrosonaphthol	p-Hydroxylated phenolic acids and 5-hydroxyindoles	Orange-red color occurs in tyrosinemia. Typical or atypical positive reactions are seen in patients with severe hepatocellular dysfunction, intestinal malabsorption or short gut syndrome, neuroblastoma, or carcinoid tumor, and in patients receiving parenteral nutrition containing N-acetyltyrosine
Merckoquant Sulfite Test	Sulfite	A pink color on the reagent strip occurs in sulfite oxidase deficiency or molybdenum cofactor defect. The reaction is inhibited by large amounts of ascorbic acid. The presence of excessive amounts of other inorganic anions and some cations produces atypical positive reactions
Benedict's reagent (Clinitest)	Reducing substances	Green to orange colors occur in glycosuria (e.g., glucose, galactose, fructose, lactose, mannose, sialic acid or xylose, but not sucrose). Homogentisic acid also produces a positive reaction. The presence of large amounts of ascorbic acid or ampicillin may interfere with the test
Acetest	Acetoacetate or acetone	Purple color indicates the presence of acetoacetate
p-Nitroaniline-nitrite reagent	Methylmalonic acid	An emerald green color indicates increased methylmalonic acid. Malonic and ethylmalonic acids, and some drugs used in pediatrics, also produce positive reactions

Note: Abbreviations: MSUD, maple syrup urine disease; PKU, phenylketonuria.

Table 9.4. *Staining reactions used for the detection and identification of amino acids in blood and urine.*

Staining reagent	Amino acids and other compounds
Ninhydrin	All amino acids
Isatin reagent (acetone/acetic acid)	Proline and hydroxyproline
Ehrlich reagent (*p*-dimethylaminobenzaldehyde)	Tryptophan and other indoles Citrulline and homocitrulline when combined with ninhydrin staining
Pauly reagent (diazotized sulfanilic acid)	Histidine, carnosine, and other imidazoles Various phenolic compounds Hydroxyproline
Sakaguchi reagent (oxine/bromine)	Arginine and other substituted guanidine compounds
Platinic iodide reagent	Sulfur-containing amino acids
Fast blue reagent (tetrazotized *o*-dianisidine)	Methylmalonic and ethylmalonic acids Phenylpyruvic acid Branched-chain keto acids

acid metabolism. The amino acid abnormality in plasma or urine may be wrongly interpreted as evidence that the underlying disease is a primary disorder of amino acid metabolism. A reasonable approach to the interpretation of plasma or urinary amino acid abnormalities might consist in addressing the following questions:

- Is the amino acid abnormality sufficiently characteristic that, along with the clinical findings in the patient, the diagnosis of a specific inborn error of metabolism can be made? This applies particularly to inborn errors of specific amino acids in which marked increases in plasma and urine levels are observed (Table 9.5).
- Is the abnormality attributable to an inherited amino acid transport abnormality? Amino acid transport abnormalities in general are characterized by markedly increased levels in urine, owing to defective reabsorption of the amino acids, along with normal or subnormal levels in plasma. The urinary amino acid pattern may be specific enough to suggest the diagnosis (Table 9.6).
- To what extent might the abnormalities be due to inherited metabolic diseases in which the disturbances in amino acid concentrations are secondary (Table 9.7)?

Table 9.5. *Plasma amino acid abnormalities in various primary disorders of amino acid metabolism.*

Amino acid abnormality	Disease (defect)	Associated clinical features
Asparrylglucosamine	Asparrylglucosaminuria	Progressive psychomotor retardation with 'storage syndrome' (Chapter 7)
Alanine	Nonspecific manifestation of lactic acidosis	
β-Alanine, taurine, GABA	Hyper-β-alaninemia Carnosinemia	Severe, early-onset neurologic syndrome with intractible seizures
α-Aminoadipic acid (2-ketoadipic acid, 2-hydroxyadipic acid)	α-Aminoadipic aciduria	Hypotonia, intermittent metabolic acidosis, developmental delay in some patients
β-Aminoisobutyric acid	β-Aminoisobutyric aciduria	Benign polymorphism; also occurs secondary to massive tissue destruction (e.g., burns, malignancy, etc.)
Anserine (β-alanyl-1-methylhistidine)	Carnosinemia	Psychomotor retardation, myoclonic seizures
Arginine	Hyperargininemia	Psychomotor retardation, spasticity resembling cerebral palsy
Argininosuccinic acid	Argininosuccinic aciduria	Hyperammonemic encephalopathy (Chapter 2)
Carnosine (β-alanylhistidine)	Carnosinemia	Psychomotor retardation, myoclonic seizures
Citrulline	Citrullinemia	Hyperammonemic encephalopathy (Chapter 2)
Cystathionine	Cystathioninemia (γ-cystathionase deficiency)	Uncertain, may be benign
Cysteine-homocysteine disulfide	Homocystinuria	See below
Glutamine	Nonspecific manifestation of hyperammonemia	
Glycine	Nonketotic hyperglycinemia (glycine cleavage deficiency)	Severe, early-onset acute encephalopathy, seizures, profound mental retardation. Glycine is also markedly increased in patients with organic acidemias, e.g., MMA, PA, IVA
Histidine	Histidinemia (histidase deficiency)	Probably benign
Homocysteine	Homocystinuria (cystathionine β-synthetase deficiency)	Psychomotor retardation, Marfanoid habitus, ectopia lentis, intravascular thrombosis (Chapter 7)
	Homocystinuria (cobalamine defects)	Megaloblastic anemia, methylmalonic acidemia, psychomotor retardation
Hydroxylysine	Hydroxylysinemia	Possible mental retardation

Hydroxyproline	Hydroxyprolinemia (hydroxyproline oxidase deficiency)	Psychomotor retardation
Leucine, isoleucine, valine	MSUD	Acute encephalopathy (Chapter 2)
Lysine	Persistent hyperlysinemia (α-aminoadipic semialdehyde synthetase deficiency)	Psychomotor retardation, seizures
Methionine	Homocystinuria (cystathionine β-synthetase deficiency)	See above
Ornithine	HHH syndrome	Recurrent hyperammonemic encephalopathy
	Hyperornithinemia with gyrate atrophy (ornithine aminotransferase deficiency)	Progressive visual impairment
Phenylalanine	Phenylketonuria	Progressive psychomotor retardation (Chapter 3)
Phosphoethanolamine	Hypophosphatasia	Skeletal dysplasia
Proline	Hyperprolinemia, type 1 (proline oxidase deficiency)	Benign
	Hyperprolinemia, type II (Δ^1-pyrroline-5-carboxylate dehydrogenase deficiency)	Seizures, relatively benign
Sarcosine (N-methylglycine)	Hypersarcosinemia	Probably benign
S-sulfocysteine	Sulfite oxidase deficiency and molybdenum cofactor deficiency	Severe, neurologic syndrome with seizures, psychomotor retardation, ectopia lentis
Tyrosine	Hereditary tyrosinemia, type I (hepatorenal tyrosinemia; fumarylacetoacetase deficiency)	Severe, progressive hepatocellular dysfunction, renal tubular dysfunction, porphyric crises (Chapter 5)
	Hereditary tyrosinemia, type II (oculocutaneous tyrosinemia; tyrosine aminotransferase deficiency)	Painful hyperkeratosis of palms and soles, painful inflammation of the eyes, corneal opacities, variable psychomotor retardation
	Hereditary tyrosinemia, type III (p-hydroxyphenylpyruvate dioxygenase deficiency)	Probably benign

Note: Abbreviations: GABA, γ-aminobutyric acid; MMA, methylmalonic acidemia; PA, propionic acidemia; IVA, isovaleric acidemia; MSUD, maple syrup urine disease; HHH, hyperornithinemia-hyperammonemia-homocitrullinemia.

Table 9.6. *Primary inherited disorders of amino acid transport.*

Amino acid abnormality	Disease (defect)	Associated clinical features
Increased cystine, arginine, lysine, ornithine, glutamine in urine	Cystinuria (defect in dibasic amino acid and cystine transport in kidney and gut)	Kidney stones, recurrent renal colic
Increased urine concentrations and decreased plasma levels of ornithine, lysine, arginine, glutamine	Lysinuric protein intolerance (generalized defect in diamino acid transport)	Dietary protein intolerance, recurrent hyperammonemia, hematologic abnormalities, pulmonary and renal disease
Increased plasma levels of ornithine, homocitrulline	HHH syndrome (defect in intramitochondrial ornithine transport)	Recurrent hyperammonemic encephalopathy (Chapter 2)
Increased urine concentrations and decreased plasma levels of neutral amino acids	Hartnup disease (defect in neutral amino acid transport in kidney and gut)	Pellagra-like skin lesions, ataxia (Chapter 2)
Increased urine concentrations of glycine, proline, hydroxyproline	Iminoglycinuria (defect in renal transport)	Benign

Note: Abbreviation: HHH, hyperammonemia-hyperornithinemia-homocitrullinemia.

Table 9.7. *Some common secondary abnormalities of plasma or urinary amino acids.*

Amino acid	Underlying condition or disease
Increased plasma alanine	Lactic acidosis, irrespective of the cause
β-Aminoisobutyric aciduria	Marked tissue destruction (burns, leukemia, surgery, etc.)
Generalized aminoaciduria	Proximal renal tubular dysfunction
1-Methylhistidinuria, carnosine	Derived from dietary poultry
Increased plasma methionine, tyrosine, and phenylalanine	Commonly associated with hepatocellular disease, irrespective of the cause
Methioninuria	Resulting from ingestion of D-methionine in semi-synthetic infant formulas supplemented with DL-methionine
Glycylprolinuria or prolylhydroxyprolinuria	Active bone disease
Increased plasma threonine	Ingestion of infant formulas with a high whey to casein ratio
Increased plasma cystathionine	Vitamin B_6 deficiency

In most of the primary inherited disorders of amino acid metabolism or transport, the plasma and urinary amino acid abnormalities are not subtle. Nonessential amino acid abnormalities are often secondary to other metabolic disorders or acquired conditions. Abnormalities involving more than one amino acid are more likely to be due to primary inherited metabolic disorders if the amino acids are structurally or metabolically related, such as the dibasic amino acids or neutral amino acids. Increased amino acid levels in the urine in the absence of corresponding increases in plasma levels are generally due to inherited or acquired renal transport defects.

Organic acid analysis

Organic analysis, by gas–liquid chromatography with or without mass spectrometry, has become available in most major pediatric hospitals. Although diagnostically important organic acid changes occur in a variety of physiological fluids, urine is the most easily obtained, the most commonly analyzed, and the fluid for which the most information is available with respect to the identification of pathologic abnormalities. With the spread of the application of high resolution tandem MS–MS technology to the investigation of inherited metabolic diseases, the analysis of organic acids in blood will become more accessible. Tandem MS–MS offers numerous advantages over conventional amino acid and organic acid analyses; however, the instrumentation is very expensive.

Most of the diagnostically important organic acids occurring in urine are chemically quite stable. The results of analysis are not materially affected by storage for periods of months at $-20°C$. The addition of chemical preservatives, such as thymol, is not generally necessary so long as the urine is kept frozen. Preparation for analysis includes extraction of the organic acids from the urine into an organic solvent. After extraction, the organic acids in physiologic fluids all require derivatization, which permits them to be heated to a vapor without undergoing thermal decomposition in the gas chromatograph.

A typical organic acid analysis would involve preliminary measurement of the creatinine concentration and dilution of a volume of urine containing 2.5 μmol to 1.0 ml with distilled water. After acidification and extraction into ethylacetate, the solvent is evaporated off, and the trimethylsilyl derivatives of the organic acids in the residue are formed immediately prior to injection into the GC–MS. The gas chromatograph is comprised of three parts: a heated inlet, a glass or steel column containing a finely ground solid support coated with a microscopic film of nonvolatile liquid phase, and a detector. The detector is often a mass spectrometer. The sample, dissolved in an appropriate solvent, is injected into the inlet where it is vaporized by heating. The vapor is carried through the column by a stream of inert gas. The compounds in the sample are separated from each other on the basis of their relative solubilities in the stationary liquid phase. Preliminary identification of organic acids is based on retention time, that is the time taken for the compound to pass through the column.

The mass spectrometer part of the system also consists of three components: a system for ionizing the compounds to be analyzed, a system for separating them on the basis of the ratio of mass to charge (m/z), and a detector. Most instruments used for clinical purposes are designed to receive the effluent from a gas chromatograph. The compounds in the effluent are ionized, commonly by bombardment by a stream of electrons, which also causes orderly fragmentation of the compounds into derivative ions of specific m/z. They are then propelled into the separating system by application of high voltage. The separating system consists of a magnetic field, most commonly produced by an array of electrodes (quadrupole) or a large magnet (magnetic sector), and the intensity of the field is varied electronically so that at any given instant only ions with a specific m/z ratio reach the detector. The detector simply records the impact of negatively charged ions as they emerge from the separator and reports the relative abundance of the ions and the m/z ratio. Compounds are identified, with the aid of computer-assisted data analysis, on the basis of a combination of retention time (gas chromatograph) and m/z and fragmentation pattern (mass spectrometer).

Primary disorders of organic acid metabolism are reviewed in detail in Chapter 4. Chemical and biological artifacts are common in the analysis of urinary organic acids. The plasticizers in plastic containers may leach out, in the presence of urine, and produce spurious signals identified as unusual fatty acids, such as azelaic and pimelic acids. Age, drugs, and diet also affect urinary organic acid profiles. Gut bacteria produce large amounts of organic acids, particularly in the very young. Some of the more common causes of urinary organic acid artifacts are shown in Table 4.8.

Acylcarnitines and acylglycines

Analysis of carnitine and glycine esters has become an important part of the investigation of organic acidopathies. Sample preparation is much easier, and the results obtained, using fast-atom bombardment (FAB) and high resolution mass spectrometry, are more powerful than conventional GC–MS. However, the capital cost of the required instrumentation puts this out of range of most diagnostic laboratories. The sensitivity of acylcarnitine analysis for the detection of inborn errors of organic acid metabolism is increased when it is combined with carnitine loading. The patient is given an oral dose of 100 mg L-carnitine per kg body weight. Urine is then collected for 8–12 hours and submitted for acylcarnitine analysis. This is sometimes necessary because carnitine levels in patients with organic acidopathies may become so depleted that there is not enough available to form diagnostic carnitine esters.

General approaches to metabolic investigation

Cellular metabolic screening studies

A number of specialized laboratories now offer metabolic screening studies based on analysis of the metabolism of specific, radiolabeled, substrates by intact cells in culture. Although simple in principle, these are generally cumbersome and require fastidious laboratory technique to produce reliable, interpretable, results. Some examples include:

- *Screening for fatty acid oxidation defects by analysis of the release of $[^{14}C]CO_2$ from radiolabeled fatty acid or organic acid substrates incubated with intact cultured skin fibroblasts.* The principle here is straight-forward; however, the application has proved to be technically demanding and for practical purposes restricted to a handful of research laboratories with special expertise in the area. When cultured fibroblasts are incubated *in situ* with $[^{14}C]$-labeled fatty acids, oxidation of the substrates results in the production of $[^{14}C]CO_2$ which is

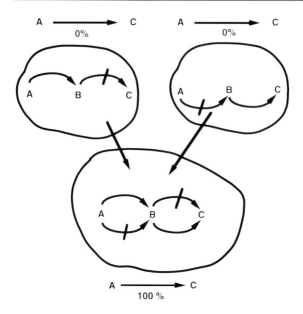

Fig. 9.1. Schematic diagram showing principles of complementation analysis.

easily trapped by concentrated NaOH or KOH. By the use of labeled fatty acid substrates of differing chain length, the relative efficiency of short-chain, medium-chain, and long-chain fatty acid oxidation can be determined. However, interpretation of the results may be difficult owing to the overlap in substrate specificities of the various enzyme systems involved in fatty acid oxidation. Selective inactivation of specific fatty acyl-CoA dehydrogenases, by precipitation with monospecific antibodies, greatly improves the diagnostic power of the technique. Identification of a presumptive defect generally requires confirmation by specific enzyme analysis.

• *Complementation testing.* Complementation analysis has been widely used to demonstrate the genetic heterogeneity of conditions which may resemble each other very closely, but are the result of mutations in different genes with gene products that are mutually complementing. The principles involved in genetic complementation analysis are illustrated diagrammatically in Figure 9.1.

Rosenblatt and others have developed elegant techniques for classifying hereditary defects in cobalamin metabolism by complementation analysis, a standard tool used in the analysis of the genetics of simple organisms, such as yeast. This involves analysis of combinations of fibroblasts cell lines, from different patients, fused together to produce hybrids in which the enzymic defect in one cell line may be corrected (i.e., complemented) by the presence of normal enzyme in the other. Cross-correction (complementation) only occurs if the defect in the two cell lines is different and either the enzymes involved, or their substrates, are freely diffusible. The analysis in this example involves incubation of various combinations of fused mutant fibroblast cell lines with radiolabeled propionic acid and determination of the extent of incorporation of label into protein. In the course of the normal metabolism of propionic acid, propionate is converted into methylmalonate, and the carbon skeleton of the methylmalonate becomes incorporated into various nonessential amino acids, which are then incorporated into protein. The classification of mutations affecting methylmalonic acid metabolic is achieved by determining the extent to which a defect observed in one cell line is corrected by fusion of the cells with cells from an individual with another genetic defect in cobalamin metabolism.

- *Testing for deficiency of one of the sphingolipid activator proteins, or for pseudodeficiency of lysosomal enzyme activities, by measuring the hydrolysis of radiolabeled, natural, substrate by intact cultured skin fibroblasts in situ.* Most of the lysosomal enzymes involved in the metabolism of sphingolipids require the presence of one of a group of nonenzymic glycoprotein activators for activity towards the natural substrate. When the activities of these enzymes are measured *in vitro*, using the natural substrates, the presence of the detergents used to maintain the substrates in aqueous solution obviates the need for the presence of a nonenzymic activator. In order to identify mutations involving one of the activator proteins, enzyme activity must be measured *in vitro* using the natural substrate, *without* any added detergent. One way to do this is to suspend radiolabeled substrate in buffer as a micellar suspension and layer this on a confluent monolayer of cultured skin fibroblasts still adherent to the base of the tissue culture dish. After several hours of incubation at 37°C, the medium is decanted, the cells are washed and harvested, and radiolabeled lipids are extracted and analyzed. The distribution of radioactivity between the labeled substrate and product reflects the activator-dependent enzyme activity.
- *Screening for defects in NADH oxidation by analysis of lactate/pyruvate (L/P) ratios in cultured skin fibroblasts.* This procedure exploits the fact that the intracellular, lactate dehydrogenase-catalyzed, interconversion of lactate and pyruvate reaches thermodynamic equilibrium so rapidly that the L/P ratio is a direct reflection of the intracellular NADH/NAD$^+$ ratio. Defects causing increased NADH concentrations are associated with increased L/P ratios, one

of the principal characteristics of mitochondrial electron transport chain defects.

- *Screening for defects in the mitochondrial ETC by culturing fibroblasts in medium containing galactose as the sole source of carbohydrate.* As a result of their impaired capacity for the production of energy from mitochondrial NADH oxidation, fibroblasts from patients with mitochondrial ETC defects rely heavily on glycolysis to meet their energy needs. When the energy-generating efficiency of glycolysis is decreased by substituting galactose for glucose in the growth medium, the viability of the cells is compromised. Whereas fibroblasts with intact mitochondrial ETC survive in galactose-containing medium, those with mitochondrial ETC defects die. Cells that fail to survive in galactose-containing medium are subjected to more detailed biochemical analysis to identify the specific ETC defect.

Provocative testing

Diagnostic tolerance tests are based on the notion that increasing the flux through a metabolic pathway which is impaired as a result of a defect in one of the specific enzymatic steps produces an increase in the concentration of the immediately proximate substrate of the defective reaction without producing an increase in the concentration of the product of the reaction. The ratio of substrate to product is increased, and normally minor metabolites often appear in easily measurable quantities. Tolerance tests are useful for evaluating, by one procedure, the integrity of an entire metabolic pathway in which equilibration between different subcellular compartmentation is not rate-limiting. Metabolic flux may be increased by:

- exogenous administration of one of the substrates of the pathway under investigation, such as phenylalanine loading for detection of carriers of PKU;
- physiologic manipulation of flux, such as by prolonged fasting, by exercise, etc.;
- exogenous hormone administration, such as administration of glucagon to test the integrity of glycogenolysis or gluconeogenesis.

Loading tests

The number of ways for evaluating the integrity of various metabolic pathways by administering supranormal amounts of one or more of the intermediates is limited only by the imagination of the investigator. However, the reliability of the testing may be limited by problems of absorption, slow equilibration among different subcellular compartments, and potential toxicity of the test metabolite. All loading tests are attended by some risk to the patient, particularly if the symptoms of disease, as is common, are attributable to accumulation of the substrate of the defective reaction. In some cases, such as fructose loading for the diagnosis of hereditary fructose intolerance, the risk of morbidity is high. Once commonly used in an effort to localize metabolic defects, metabolic loading tests are now rarely used to screen for genetic defects of intermediary metabolism. This is partly because tolerance tests are dangerous. In most cases, analysis of the specific enzyme presumed to be involved in the defect is available, it is much more specific, and it is safer.

Physiologic stress tests

Closely monitored, controlled starvation is one of the most common stress tests employed to assess the physiologic response to fasting. During the transition from the fed to the fasting state, important adjustments in the body to ensure an adequate continuing supply of energy to vital organs, like the brain, while minimizing the mobilization of energy substrates from tissues like muscle protein.

A typical test for the evaluation of the efficiency of mitochondrial fatty acid oxidation takes up to 24 hours, depending on the age of the patient and the history of tolerance of fasting (see Chapter 5). Fasting is generally begun in the early evening with occasional biochemical monitoring during the night. On the following morning, a slowly running intravenous of 0.9% NaCl is established to facilitate blood sampling and the rapid administration of glucose should the need arise. After obtaining blood and urine for baseline analysis of glucose, 3-hydroxybutyrate and acetoacetate, free fatty acids, and carnitine (free and total), in plasma, and ketones (by Acetest; Ames), organic acids, carnitine (free and total), acylcarnitines, and acylglycines, in urine, the blood glucose is monitored hourly until the patient develops symptoms of hypoglycemia, or until 20 hours has elapsed, whichever comes first. All urine passed should be tested for ketones. At the termination of the fast, blood and urine are again obtained for the same studies done at baseline. If the patient is symptomatic or hypoglycemic by finger-prick monitoring, the test blood sample should be obtained without delay and the patient given glucose by intravenous infusion until asymptomatic and stable.

The normal response to fasting includes a gradual fall in plasma glucose, rise in plasma ketones (3-hydroxybutyrate and acetoacetate), rise in plasma free fatty acids, and the appearance of ketones and small quantities of medium-chain dicarboxylic acids in the urine. The ratio of free fatty acids to 3-hydroxybutyrate normally does not exceed 3.0. Patients with fatty acid oxidation defects often become hypoglycemic during this procedure, but the ketone levels in plasma do not rise significantly, resulting in a marked elevation of the free fatty acid to 3-hydroxybutyrate ratio. Analysis of urinary organic acids, acylcarnitines, and acylglycines shows the presence of intermediates typical of the underlying defect.

Hormone stimulation tests

Glucagon stimulation is an excellent way to evaluate the integrity of glycogenolysis and gluconeogenesis. However, accurate interpretation of the results requires careful preparation of the patient. For example, the absence of a glycemic response to intramuscular administration of an appropriate dose of the hormone after several hours of fasting may be the result of a defect in glycogen mobilization, such as glycogen debranching enzyme deficiency, or to prior depletion of liver glycogen by prolonged starvation (see Chapter 5).

Enzymology

A strong presumptive diagnosis of a specific inherited metabolic condition is often possible on the basis of the results of analysis of the substrates and products of a particular enzymic reaction, and awareness of the significance of various secondary metabolic abnormalities. This is particularly true of defects in the metabolism of water soluble metabolites, such as amino acids. The abnormalities of amino acid concentrations in maple syrup urine disease are so typical, for example, that specific analysis of branched-chain 2-ketoacid dehydrogenase activity in tissues is generally not diagnostically necessary, except of course in the case of prenatal diagnosis. Analysis of specific defects in amino acid transport is rarely necessary to make the diagnosis of various transport defects, such as dibasic amino aciduria, lysinuric protein intolerance, cystinosis, or hyperammonemia-hyperornithinemia-homocitrullinemia, which are all identifiable by the effects the defects have on the concentration of water-soluble metabolites in plasma, urine, and tissues.

However, the definitive diagnosis of many other inherited metabolic diseases is not possible without the demonstration of specific deficiency of the enzyme involved. Prenatal diagnosis, in particular, requires access to specific enzyme assays, or to DNA analysis in cases in which the diagnosis of the disease under investigation is established and the specific mutations, or appropriate linkage markers, are known. Reliance on the measurement of specific enzyme activities for diagnosis, including prenatal diagnosis, requires awareness of the normal tissue distribution of the relevant enzymes and their stability.

The practical application of clinical diagnostic enzymology demands attention to a number of variables affecting the results of any particular assay. Although the details of the conditions for measurement of specific enzyme activities vary tremendously from one enzyme to another, the nature of the variables is the same for any diagnostically important enzyme. They include:

- *The source of the enzyme to be assayed (tissue specificity)*. 'House-keeping' enzymes are widely distributed in the body, and the selection of the tissue or fluid most suitable for analysis of activity is often based on accessibility, plasma or urine being the most accessible, and brain being relatively inaccessible. Some enzymes are tissue specific, and diagnostic analysis requires sampling of the relevant tissue.
- *The stability of the enzyme*. Most enzymes, like most proteins, are very sensitive to storage conditions, and storage under suboptimal conditions leads to losses of enzyme activity which might confound the interpretation of test results. However, other enzymes are very stable; they will withstand drying on filter paper and storage at room temperature for extended periods of time. In general, most enzymes can be stored frozen in tissue at –70°C virtually indefinitely without loss of activity.
- *The reaction conditions*. It goes without saying that the assay conditions used for the analysis of enzyme activities should be optimum for the measurement of the rate of enzyme-catalyzed conversion substrate to product. This includes the selection of a suitable buffer system, pH, ionic strength, and substrate concentration, as well as the temperature, protein concentration, and incubation time used. As a rule, enzyme activities analyzed for clinical diagnostic purposes are measured under conditions that produce zero-order enzyme kinetics. That is, the conditions are selected to ensure that the rate of conversion of substrate to product is directly proportional to the amount of enzyme present.
- *The substrate specificity of the enzyme*. Most enzymes are extremely fastidious with respect to substrate preference, extending even to specificity for particular optical isomers of substrate compounds. However, in some cases, particularly in the diagnosis of diseases due to defects of lysosomal enzyme activities, advantage is taken of the relatively relaxed substrate specificity of the enzymes for the easy demonstration of enzyme deficiencies. This is reviewed in somewhat greater detail in the section below on lysosomal disorders.
- *The influence of metabolic regulators on activity*. Some enzymes require the presence of specific metabolic effectors for optimum activity. In some cases, these compounds are cosubstrates in the reaction and variations in their concentration or omission from the assay mixture has profound effects on the

activity of the enzyme under investigation. In other cases, the effect of metabolic effectors is more complex: they may serve as allosteric activators which significantly alter the enzyme kinetics in a non-linear fashion. In general, the activity of allosteric enzymes is best assessed for clinical purposes under reaction conditions which produce maximum enzyme activity.

The activities of some enzymes are profoundly affected by enzyme-catalyzed modification, such as phosphorylation, of the enzyme itself. The activities of some of the rate-limiting enzymes involved in glucose metabolism, such as hepatic phosphorylase and pyruvate dehydrogenase (PDH), exhibit this characteristic. In one case (phosphorylase), the activity of the enzyme is increased by phosphorylation catalyzed by a specific kinase; in the other (PDH), phosphorylation by the relevant specific PDH kinase inhibits enzyme activity. In both situations, specific phosphatases reverse the changes in activity produced by phosphorylation. Each of the enzymes is encoded by a different gene under independent genetic control. Complete characterization of this type of enzyme system for clinical diagnostic purposes calls for measurements under different reaction conditions, including under ambient and fully activated conditions.

- *Developmental changes in enzyme activities.* The activities of some enzymes, such as plasma alkaline phosphatase, vary significantly with age. The interpretation of the results of any measurements must be done on the basis of age-related normal values.

- *The phenomenon of 'pseudodeficiency'.* A number of situations have been identified in which apparently completely healthy individuals were found to have marked deficiency of the activity of a particular enzyme, as measured *in vitro* under normal assay conditions. This phenomenon of pseudodeficiency is particularly common among the lysosomal hydrolases and has the potential to produce major diagnostic confusion.

Molecular genetic studies

Clinicians are relying increasingly on molecular genetic studies to confirm the diagnosis of genetic disease, including genetic metabolic diseases. The availability of specific molecular genetic testing is expanding rapidly, though there remain some serious limitations on the general diagnostic use of the methodology.

There is no question that the techniques currently available for the detection of specific mutations are technically relatively simple, and the results are generally unambiguous: either the mutation is present or it is not. If homozygosity for the mutation is known to cause a particular disease, then the demonstration of two copies of the mutant allele is virtually diagnostic of the condition. However, the power of the approach is diluted by the problem of *allelic diversity*.

With very few exceptions, in all inherited metabolic diseases for which the responsible gene has been isolated and disease-producing mutations characterized, no single mutation accounts for all cases of the disease. Instead, the mutations associated with each disease usually number in the dozens with single specific mutations accounting for no more than a simple majority of the mutant alleles. What this means in practical terms is that while the detection of a certain mutation in tissue from a patient is generally considered strong support for the diagnosis of the related disease, the failure to demonstrate the presence of the mutation, or even a number of different mutations in the same gene, does not rule out the diagnosis. The patient may simply have mutations that have not yet been characterized. But, in certain cases, and within some specific ethnic groups, the number of different alleles accounting for a high proportion of the cases of a particular disease may be small enough to enable strong diagnostic inferences to be made on the basis of molecular genetic analysis. The absence of specific mutant alleles should always be interpreted with care: the disease in any specific individual may be caused by a mutation that has not previously been identified with the disorder. In such cases, the analysis of the gene product, by measurement of enzyme activity, for example, is a more powerful test of the presence of disease-causing mutations in the relevant gene. Some conditions in which specific mutant alleles occur with sufficient frequency in selected populations to be useful diagnostically are shown in Table 9.8.

A number of techniques have been developed to screen specific genes for sequence abnormalities. Southern blot analysis is useful for the detection of significant deletions or insertions or for sequence changes producing new restriction sites or deleting restriction sites present in the normal gene. Other techniques, such as chemical cleavage and single strand conformation polymorphism (SSCP) analysis, are sensitive, but they are technically cumbersome. Moreover, additional genetic and molecular studies are necessary to prove that any sequence change that is discovered is not simply a harmless polymorphism. Despite current technical difficulties, diagnosis by molecular analysis is growing very rapidly.

Lysosomal disorders

Lysosomes are single-membrane subcellular organelles which contain a large number of enzymes involved in the hydrolysis of high molecular weight or water-insoluble compounds, like membranes, complex lipids, proteins, and

Table 9.8. *Some common mutations causing specific inherited metabolic diseases.*

Disease	Gene	Mutation
MCAD deficiency	MCAD	K304E
Tay-Sachs disease (Ashkenazi Jews)	HEXA	+TATC$_{1278}$[†]
Gaucher disease (Ashkenazi Jews)	GBA	N370S
α_1-Antitrypsin deficiency	PI*Z	E342K
LCHAD deficiency	LCHAD (α-subunit)	E510Q
Galactosemia	GALT	Q188R
MPS IH	IDUA	W402X
LHON	ND4	G11778A[†]
PKU	PAH	R408W

Note: Abbreviations: MCAD, medium-chain acyl-CoA dehydrogenase; LCHAD, long-chain 3-hydroxyacyl-CoA dehydrogenase; MPS IH, Hurler disease; LHON, Lebers hereditary optic neuropathy; PKU, phenylketonuria.
[†] Nucleotide change.

nucleic acids, derived either from the normal turnover of intracellular structures or from similar materials taken up from the extracellular environment by endocytosis/phagocytosis. Lysosomal hydrolases are glycoproteins which become localized in lysosomes by virtue of modification of the oligosaccharide part of the enzyme molecule to contain a mannose-phosphate signal moiety, which is subsequently removed inside the lysosome. Defects in the synthesis of this signal moiety cause I-cell disease, a condition characterized by failure of lysosomal enzymes to become localized within lysosomes. Some lysosomal enzymes, like most of the sphingolipid hydrolases, require the presence of genetically distinct, non-catalytic, activator proteins for activity against their natural substrates. Disease resulting from mutations affecting activator proteins is clinically indistinguishable from that caused by deficiency of the respective lysosomal enzyme. Other lysosomal enzymes, such as α-neuraminidase and β-galactosidase, require the presence of a protective protein to prevent premature breakdown. Mutations affecting production of the protective protein cause combined deficiency of both enzymes and a disease called galactosialidosis.

Most of this class of enzymes exhibits relatively relaxed substrate specificity. Lysosomal hydrolases, with some important exceptions, are highly specific for the leaving group of the reaction. As a group, the glycosidases are specific for the monosaccharide removed from the substrate glycoconjugate; they are also very specific for the anomeric configuration of the glycosidic linkage, α or β. In contrast, they are not as fastidious with regard to the specific structure of the aglycone, the non-carbohydrate part of the molecule. Accordingly, the lysosomal enzyme, β-galactosidase, which catalyzes the hydrolysis of the galactose residue from the non-reducing end of the oligosaccharide of the sphingolipid, GM1 ganglioside, is very specific for an unsubstituted galactose in β-anomeric glycosidic linkage to the rest of the substrate molecule, the aglycone. However, a large number of compounds can be substituted for the aglycone for the purposes of the measurement of β-galactosidase activity. When the substituting aglycone is a relatively simple, water-soluble, chromogenic or fluorogenic compound, the measurement of enzyme activity becomes easy: the rate of enzyme-catalyzed hydrolysis of the synthetic, 'artificial', substrate is measured by the change in absorbance or fluorescence at specific wavelengths depending on the nature of the aglycone. Lysosomes have an acid pH, and the pH optima of all lysosomal hydrolases, regardless of the substrate, is in the acid range (pH 4.5–6.0).

The laboratory investigation of diseases caused by hereditary deficiency of lysosomal enzymes involves three sorts of studies of increasing specificity and sophistication:

- morphologic studies;
- identification of the chemical nature of compounds accumulating as a result of the enzyme deficiency;
- demonstration of a specific enzyme deficiency.

Morphologic studies

Many lysosomal storage diseases are characterized by the presence of morphologic changes identifiable on radiographs of bones (see Chapter 7), or on histologic, histochemical, or electron microscopic studies on tissues obtained by biopsy. One of the simplest tests is microscopic examination of a routine Wright-stained peripheral blood smear for the presence of metachromatic granules (Alder-Reilly bodies) in monocytes and large lymphocytes (Figure 7.3), which is a feature of many, though not all, mucopolysaccharide storage diseases. However, although the test is inexpensive and widely available, the differentiation of Alder-Reilly bodies from other types of inclusions requires some experience, and failure to demonstrate their presence does not eliminate the possibility of an MPS disorder.

Bone marrow is also a readily accessible tissue which often shows diagnostically significant morphologic changes in patients with lysosomal storage diseases. In some cases, like Gaucher disease, the morphology of the storage cell is

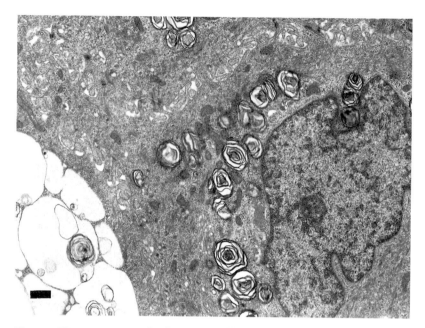

Fig. 9.2. Electron micrograph of conjunctival biopsy in mucolipidosis type IV showing fibrillogranular flocculent material (lower left) and abundant membranous lammellar bodies. The bar represents 1 μm. (Courtesy of Dr. Venita Jay.)

sufficiently characteristic that a strong presumptive diagnosis can be made on the basis of these findings alone (see Figure 7.5).

Conjunctival biopsy is technically simple, and coupled with electron microscopic examination it provides important, often diagnostic, information in patients with neurodegenerative lysosomal disorders, such as neuronal ceroid lipofuscinosis (see Figure 2.2) and mucolipidosis type IV (Figure 9.2). It is generally just as informative and less invasive than rectal or brain biopsy.

Biopsies of brain or nerve, or of parenchymatous organs, like liver, are rarely required for the diagnosis of lysosomal diseases. On the one hand, the pathologic changes are rarely specific enough to make a diagnosis that could not be made biochemically or by biopsy of more accessible tissues. On the other hand, if tissue is available, histochemical and ultrastructural studies may provide guidance for further more definitive studies.

Identification of accumulating compounds (storage material)

In general, studies on the structural analysis of stored compounds sufficiently sophisticated to suggest a specific enzyme deficiency are rarely practical in the clinical diagnosis of lysosomal storage disorders. The amount of tissue required is too large to be obtainable before death, and the analytic studies required to establish the structure of the stored material are generally available only in research laboratories with a special interest in this class of disorders. With some idea of the class of compound involved, derived from the results of morphologic investigation and some relatively unsophisticated biochemical tests, such as the urinary MPS screening test discussed below, the specific enzyme defect can be identified with a fraction of the effort by assaying several enzymes in a suitable tissue, such as leukocytes or fibroblasts.

Urinary mucopolysaccharide (MPS) tests

There are many screening tests for excess acidic mucopolysaccharide in urine; almost all of them are based on tests for the presence of increased amounts of high molecular weight polyanions in urine. This may involve precipitation of the compounds, by addition of a detergent, with the production of turbidity, or a change in the color of a metachromatic dye, such as toluidine blue or Alcian blue. Various laboratory test manufacturers have developed methods to simplify testing, such as impregnating a metachromatic dye in paper. Only a few drops of urine are required, and the test takes only seconds to perform. The sensitivity of all MPS screening tests is high. However, false positives are very common, particularly in young infants. False negatives also occur, particularly in patients with Morquio disease (MPS IV) and less often in Sanfilippo disease (MPS III).

The amount of MPS in urine can be estimated by measuring the turbidity of a urine specimen after addition of a detergent which precipitates the compounds, or by quantitating spectrophotometrically the amount of Alcian blue dye bound by precipitated MPS. Thin-layer chromatographic analysis (TLC) of urinary MPS is more cumbersome, but it provides information important to the classification of the disorder by indicating the relative proportions of dermatan sulfate, heparan sulfate, keratan sulfate, and chondroitin sulfate (Table 9.9).

Urinary oligosaccharide analysis

Oligosaccharides are low molecular weight carbohydrate polymers made up of at least three monosaccharide subunits. The oligosaccharides in urine are derived from the incomplete breakdown of the carbohydrate side-chains of complex glycoproteins. The structures of the excreted compounds reflect the carbohydrate composition of the oligosaccharide and the role that various lysosomal enzymes play in their metabolism (Figure 9.3).

TLC of unconcentrated urine is the most widely employed method for screening for the glycoproteinoses (Chapter 7). Only a very small aliquot of urine

Table 9.9. *Urinary MPS in the different mucopolysaccharidoses (MPS).*

Disease	Dermatan sulfate	Heparan sulfate	Keratan sulfate	Chondroitin sulfate
MPS I	++++	+	−	+
MPS II	+++	+	−	+
MPS III	−	+++	−	+
MPS IV	−	−	++	+
MPS VI	+++	±	−	+
MPS VII	++	±	−	++*
Normal	±	±	±	+

Note: *Reported early in the course of some cases of the disease.

(≤ 0.5 ml) is needed for the analysis. The amount of urine spotted for TLC is adjusted to correspond to a constant amount of creatinine to obviate the need for 24-hour collections of urine. Urine specimens require no preservative, but they should be stored frozen at $-20°C$ until analyzed.

Unfortunately, this relatively inexpensive screening test is not particularly sensitive, and the specificity is also low. Patients with GM1 gangliosidosis, galactosialidosis, sialidosis, or Schindler disease are rarely missed; the urinary oligosaccharide analysis is generally obvious. On the other hand, the excretion of oligosaccharides by patients with other glycoproteinoses is variable. The urine of patients with α-mannosidosis, α-fucosidosis, Sandhoff disease, or aspartyl-glucosaminuria usually shows increased amounts of oligosaccharides, although the abnormalities may be very subtle. Urine specimens from patients with β-mannosidosis, I-cell disease (mucolipidosis II) or pseudo-Hurler polydys-trophy (mucolipidosis III) generally do not contain excess amounts of oligosac-charides. Oligosacchariduria is a feature of some glycogen storage diseases, such as Pompe disease (GSD II), and we have seen it in some patients with Gaucher disease. Spurious oligosacchariduria occurs in patients infused with large amounts of complex carbohydrate, such as dextran. Neonates also commonly show the presence of oligosaccharide bands that would be interpreted as abnormal in older children. The cost of pursuing false positive oligosac-chariduria has been so high that some reputable laboratories have abandoned the test altogether and screen for the glycoproteinoses by testing leukocytes with batteries of several lysosomal enzyme assays. Some representative TLC analyses of urinary oligosaccharides are shown in Figure 9.4.

Structural analysis of individual oligosaccharides detected by TLC is beyond the scope of most diagnostic laboratories, and it is certainly not more cost

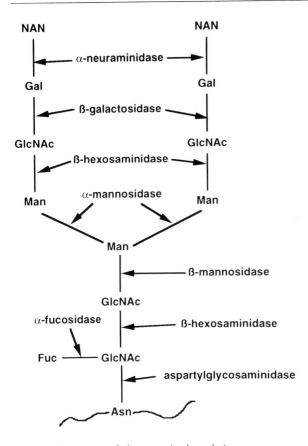

Fig. 9.3. Summary of glycoprotein degradation.

effective than simply running through all the possible glycoproteinoses by measurement of the relevant lysosomal enzyme activities in leukocytes or fibroblasts.

Demonstration of specific enzyme deficiency

Owing to the clinical similarity between various lysosomal disorders, the final diagnosis in each case rests on the ability to demonstrate a specific enzyme deficiency to account for the disease. Table 9.10 shows a summary of the enzyme defects in each of the known lysosomal enzyme deficiency diseases and the most readily accessible source of enzyme for diagnostic analysis.

Fibroblasts are probably the best material for diagnosis of lysosomal disorders by enzyme assay. However, obtaining enough cells for reliable analyses often

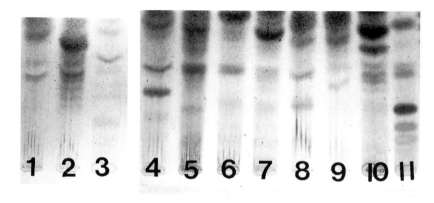

Fig. 9.4. Thin-layer chromatographic analysis of urinary oligosaccharides. The various lanes show analyses of urine from patients with different glycoproteinoses. Lane 1, Normal; 2, α-Mannosidosis; 3, α-Fucosidosis; 4, Aspartylglucosaminuria; 5, Farber lipogranulomatosis; 6, MPS IH (Hurler disease); 7, I-cell disease; 8, Galactosialidosis; 9, Glycogen storage disease, type III; 10, Glycogen storage disease, type II (Pompe disease); 11, GM1 gangliosidosis.

takes weeks in culture. The analysis of enzyme activities in leukocytes is equally reliable in some cases. In others, the presence of non-lysosomal isozymes may obscure deficiency of the lysosomal enzyme when the assay is carried out with leukocytes. For example, leukocytes contain a neutral, non-lysosomal α-glucosidase. In order to make the diagnosis of GSD II on the basis of measurements of lysosomal α-glucosidase in leukocytes, particular care must be taken to account for enzyme activity attributable to the non-lysosomal enzyme. Enzyme analysis is still the most common technique used for detection of carriers of lysosomal storage disease mutations. However, in many cases, the overlap between the enzyme activities in leukocytes from homozygous normal individuals and heterozygotes is sufficient to result in misclassification in 10–15% of carriers. The advent of molecular genetic testing for the detection of carriers by the detection of specific mutations is a major advance in genetic counselling of family members of individuals affected with lysosomal enzyme deficiency diseases.

Disorders of mitochondrial energy metabolism

Muscle is almost always involved to some extent, if not primarily, in inborn errors of mitochondrial energy metabolism (see Chapter 2). Histochemical, electron microscopic, and biochemical studies on the tissue are the principal

Table 9.10. *Summary of assays useful in the investigation of lysosomal storage diseases.*

Disease	Enzyme	Enzyme source
Mucopolysaccharide storage diseases		
Hurler disease (MPS IH)	α-L-iduronidase	L, F
Scheie disease (MPS IS)	α-L-iduronidase	L, F
Hunter disease (MPS II)	Iduronate 2-sulfatase	S, L, F
Sanfilippo disease, type A (MPS IIIA)	Heparan *N*-sulfatase	L, F
Sanfilippo disease, type B (MPS IIIB)	α-*N*-Acetylglucosaminidase	L, F
Sanfilippo disease, type C (MPS IIIC)	Acetyl-CoA:α-glucosaminide acetyltransferase	F
Sanfilippo disease, type D (MPS IIID)	*N*-Acetylglucosamine 6-sulfatase	L, F
Morquio disease, type A (MPS IVA)	*N*-Acetylgalactosamine 6-sulfatase	L, F
Morquio disease, type B (MPS IVB)	β-Galactosidase	S, L, F
Maroteaux-Lamy disease (MPS VI)	*N*-Acetylgalactosamine 4-sulfatase (arylsulfatase B)	L, F
Sly disease (MPS VII)	β-Glucuronidase	S, L, F
Mucolipidoses (Oligosaccharide storage diseases)		
Aspartylglucosaminuria	Aspartylglucosaminidase	L, F
GM1 gangliosidosis	β-Galactosidase	S, L, F
α-Mannosidosis	α-Mannosidase	L, F
β-Mannosidosis	β-Mannosidase	L, F
Sialidosis	α-Neuraminidase	F
Galactosialidosis	α-Neuraminidase and β-galactosidase	F
α-Fucosidosis	α-Fucosidase	S, L, F
Schindler disease	α-Glucosaminidase	L, F
I-Cell disease (and also mucolipidosis III, pseudo-Hurler polydystrophy)	β-Hexosaminidase	S **and** L
Sphingolipidoses		
Fabry disease	α-Galactosidase	S, L, F
Gaucher disease	Glucocerebrosidase (β-glucosidase)	L, F
Niemann-Pick disease, types A and B	Acid sphingomyelinase	L, F
Niemann-Pick disease, type C	Cholesterol esterification	F
Metachromatic leukodystrophy (MLD)	Arylsulfatase A	L, F
Krabbe globoid cell leukodystrophy	Galactocerebrosidase	L, F
Farber lipogranulomatosis	Ceramidase	L, F

Note: L, peripheral blood leukocytes; F, cultured skin fibroblasts; S, serum.

means by which definitive diagnosis is made in most cases, though studies on cultured fibroblasts are often helpful.

Morphologic studies

Lytic lesions in the basal ganglia and thalamus, sometimes extending into the midbrain, are often seen in CT and MRI scans of the CNS in patients with chronic encephalopathies associated with mitochondrial ETC defects. However, the histochemical and electron microscopic findings in skeletal muscle are perhaps the most characteristic morphologic abnormalities in patients with mutations affecting mitochondrial energy metabolism. Skeletal and cardiac muscle typically shows accumulation of lipid and glycogen. However, the changes produced by proliferation, aggregation, and distortion of mitochondria are particularly instructive. The subsarcolemmal accumulation of mitochondria produces a typical ragged-red fiber appearance when sections of the tissue are stained by the modified Gomori trichrome method. This is illustrated in Figure 2.7 where mitochondrial myopathies are discussed in somewhat more detail. Electron microscopic examination often shows distortion of the mitochondria, with abnormalities of the cristae and matrix, and accumulation of paracrystalline inclusions between the mitochondrial membranes or in the cristae.

Biochemical studies

The ultimate definition of abnormalities arising from mutations affecting mitochondrial energy metabolism rests on biochemical evaluation of mitochondrial function. The assessment of mitochondrial function *in vitro* has been advanced tremendously by:

- the development of techniques for the analysis of ETC function in lymphocytes, fibroblasts, and mitochondria isolated from very small samples of tissue, particularly muscle;
- methods for studying mitochondrial function *in situ* in lymphocytes and cultured skin fibroblasts by permeablization of the cell membrane by treatment with detergents;
- the development of monospecific antibodies for measuring the activities of different enzymes, such as the acyl-CoA dehydrogenases, with overlapping substrate specificities;
- the use of various synthetic chromogenic electron acceptors, along with specific electron transport inhibitors, to evaluate the integrity of the different multiprotein complexes of the mitochondrial ETC;
- the rapidly growing application of molecular genetic techniques to the

characterization of the various components of mitochondrial energy metabolism.

Familiarity with some of the theoretical and technical issues involved in the assessment of this very complex system makes the clinical investigation of disorders of mitochondrial energy metabolism easier to follow. Assessment of mitochondrial energy metabolism embraces five types of process, each associated with defects producing disease. Detailed analysis of most of these is available only in laboratories doing active research on disorders of energy metabolism.

Substrate transport

Most of the energy derived from fatty acid oxidation is generated by the process of β-oxidation, which takes place in the mitochondrial matrix. The transport of fatty acids into mitochondria involves the participation of four distinct gene products, two enzymes and two membrane transporters (Figure 9.5).

Fatty acids entering the cytosol are rapidly esterified to form coenzyme A derivatives. Transport into mitochondria requires transesterification with free carnitine to form fatty acylcarnitine in a reaction catalyzed by the enzyme *carnitine palmitoyltransferase I* located in the outer mitochondrial membrane. Transport of the fatty acylcarnitine through the inner mitochondrial membrane involves *carnitine-acylcarnitine translocase*, a co-transporter which facilitates transport of acylcarnitine in one direction and free carnitine in the other. Finally, the fatty acylcarnitine inside mitochondria is transesterified to regenerate long-chain fatty acyl-CoA in a reaction catalyzed by carnitine palmitoyltransferase II. The fourth gene product required for the process to work is the *carnitine transporter* in the cell membrane which, along with carnitine-acylcarnitine translocase, ensures adequate cytosolic concentrations of free carnitine to support production of fatty acylcarnitines.

Substrate utilization

Pyruvate carboxylase (PC) catalyzes the most important of the anaplerotic reactions which function to ensure the supply of tricarboxylic acid (TCA) cycle intermediates is adequate to support the cycle. It is a biotin-dependent enzyme which catalyzes the carboxylation of pyruvate to form oxaloacetate. It is dependent for activity on the presence of acetyl-CoA, an allosteric activator of the enzyme. In addition to its role in fueling the TCA cycle, PC catalyzes the first, and most important, reaction in gluconeogenesis.

PDH is a huge multicomponent enzyme complex made up of multiple units of 4 enzymes: pyruvate decarboxylase (E_1, 30 units), dihydrolipoyl transacetylase

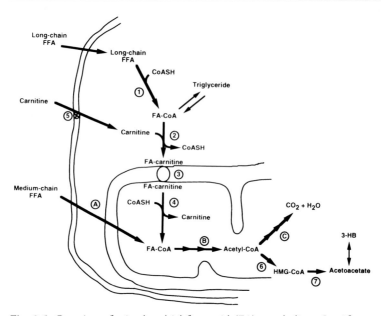

Fig. 9.5. Overview of mitochondrial fatty acid (FA) metabolism. Specific enzymes are shown here as numerals, and processes are represented by letters of the alphabet. The processes shown are: **A**, medium-chain free fatty acid (FFA) uptake and diffusion into mitochondria without activation to coenzyme A (CoA) esters; **B**, fatty acid β-oxidation; **C**, oxidation of acetyl-CoA via the tricarboxylic acid cycle. The enzymes involved in various reactions are: **1**, long-chain fatty acid:CoA ligase; **2**, carnitine palmitoyltransferase I (CPT I); **3**, carnitine:acylcarnitine translocase; **4**, carnitine palmitoyltransferase II (CPT II); **5**, transmembrane carnitine translocase; **6**, 3-hydroxy-3-methylglutaryl-CoA synthetase; **7**, 3-hydroxy-3-methylglutaryl-CoA (HMG-CoA) lyase.

(E_2, 60 units), dihydrolipoyl dehydrogenase (E_3, 6 units), and protein X (6 units). The enzyme catalyzes the oxidative decaboxylation of pyruvate to acetyl-CoA. Enzyme activity is regulated by phosphorylation (inactivation)–dephosphorylation (activation) in reactions catalyzed by PDH kinase and PDH phosphatase, respectively. It is customary when measuring PDH activity in tissue extracts to do the assay in the presence and absence of dicloroacetate, an inhibitor of PDH kinase, to determine total PDH activity and the proportion in the active form, respectively.

PC deficiency and PDH deficiency are both associated with persistent, severe, lactic acidosis (see Chapter 4). The majority of cases of PDH deficiency are the result of mutations in the X-linked α subunit of E_1. Overall, males and females are equally affected except among patients with the mildest form of the disease,

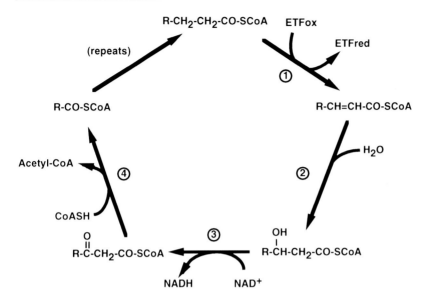

Fig. 9.6. Mitochondrial fatty acid β-oxidation.
The enzymes involved in mitochondrial fatty acid β-oxidation are: **1**, fatty acyl-CoA dehydrogenases (short-chain, medium-chain, long-chain, and very long-chain); **2**, 2-enol-CoA hydratases; **3**, L-3-hydroxyacyl-CoA dehydrogenases; **4**, 3-ketoacyl-CoA thiolases.

which is characterized by intermittent ataxia and appears only to occur in males (see Chapter 2).

Defects in fatty acid oxidation may arise as a result of mutations affecting any one of several enzymes involved in the process (see Chapter 5). The fatty acyl-CoA dehydrogenases are FAD-containing enzymes which catalyze the first step in the mitochondrial β-oxidation of fatty acids (Figure 9.6), the introduction of a *trans* double bond, and transfer of electrons from the substrate to electron transfer flavoprotein (ETF). The four genetically distinct mitochondrial fatty acyl-CoA dehydrogenases (SCAD, MCAD, LCAD, and VLCAD) differ in their substrate specificities, though there is considerable overlap between them in this regard. Long-chain 2-enoyl-CoA hydratase, 3-hydroxyacyl-CoA dehydrogenase, and 3-ketoacyl-CoA thiolase activities exist in the mitochondrion as a trifunctional protein. The corresponding short-chain substrate-specific enzymes appear to exist as separate proteins.

Analytical screening techniques have been developed to assess fatty acid oxidation *in situ* in cultured fibroblasts using [^{14}C]-labeled fatty acids and measuring the production of $^{14}CO_2$. This has been coupled with assays to identify defects in specific enzymes involved in fatty acid oxidation. The analysis of steps in fatty acid β-oxidation catalyzed by more than one enzyme with different chain-length specificities, such as the fatty acyl-CoA dehydrogenases, is complicated by overlapping substrate specificities of the enzymes. Measurement of medium-chain acyl-CoA dehydrogenase (MCAD) activity inevitably includes activity contributed by long-chain and short-chain acyl-CoA dehydrogenases (LCAD and SCAD, respectively), unless these enzymes are inactivated. This can be done by specific immunoprecipitation of the dehydrogenases contaminating the measurement of the enzyme activity of interest.

Complementation analysis is another approach to pin-pointing a defect in fatty acid oxidation. Cells with a known defect are fused with cells from the patient, and the effect on [^{14}C]fatty acid oxidation is determined. If the defect in the two cell lines is the same, fusion of the cells will have no effect on $^{14}CO_2$ production from radiolabeled substrate. But, if the defects in the two cell lines are different, they will be mutually corrected when cells from the two lines are fused.

Electron transport chain (ETC)

The mitochondrial ETC encompasses an assemblage of polypeptide gene products arranged in the mitochondrial membrane to transfer the energy derived from the oxidation of NADH and succinate to produce ATP. The process is achieved by the consecutive participation of as many as 83 polypeptides, arranged in five multicomponent complexes, Complexes I to V, through which the electrons pass to be accepted finally by O_2 to form H_2O and generate ATP (Figure 9.7). The majority of the polypeptides involved are the products of nuclear genes and cytosolic protein biosynthesis, the rest are coded by mitochondrial genes and synthesized within the mitochondrion (Table 9.11). Most of the diseases caused by nuclear gene mutations are transmitted as autosomal recessive disorders.

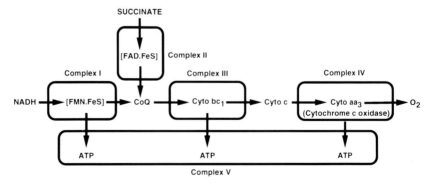

Fig. 9.7. Complexes of the mitochondrial electron transport chain.

Table 9.11. *Subunits of mitochondrial electron transport chain.*

Electron transport complex	Inhibitor	Subunits coded by	
		mtDNA	nDNA
Complex I (NADH:ubiquinone oxidoreductase)	Rotenone	7	≈ 34
Complex II (Succinate:ubiquinone oxidoreductase)		0	4
Complex III (Ubiquinol:ferrocytochrome c oxidoreductase or cytochrome bc_1 complex)	Antimycin	1	10
Complex IV (ferrocytochrome c:oxygen oxidoreductase)	Cyanide	3	10
Complex V (ATP synthase)	Oligomycin	2	11 or 12

The laboratory investigation of mitochondrial ETC defects is similar, in principle, to the investigation of fatty acid β-oxidation defects. Respiration of intact lymphocytes, fibroblasts, or isolated muscle mitochondria is assessed polarographically (i.e., by measurement of oxygen utilization) using various energy substrates and specific ETC inhibitors. ETC activity of the individual complexes is then measured spectrophotometrically. Cytochrome c oxidase (Complex IV) is measured directly by spectrophotometry. Marked deficiency of the activity of the complex can sometimes be determined histochemically. Complexes I and III are measured together by spectrophotometric analysis of rotenone-sensitive NADH-cytochrome c reductase activity. Complexes II and III are evaluated together by measurement of succinate cytochrome c reductase activity. Complex I alone is evaluated by measurement of rotenone-sensitive NADH oxidation in the presence of decyl ubiquinone as electron acceptor.

Peroxisomal disorders
Peroxisomes are single-membrane subcellular organelles which contribute both biosynthetic and catabolic functions to tissues throughout the body. Some of the key functions of peroxisomes are shown in Table 9.12.

Morphologic studies
The appearance on electron microscopy of the peroxisomes in liver obtained by biopsy is particularly informative in the investigation of peroxisomal disorders. Abnormalities in shape or number, including total absence of the organelle, are characteristic of the peroxisomal assembly defects, such as classical Zellweger syndrome. However, in many of the diseases caused by single peroxisomal enzyme deficiencies, such as X-linked adrenoleukodystrophy, peroxisomal morphology is normal.

Table 9.12. *Some key functions of peroxisomes.*

Biosynthetic processes	Catabolic processes
Synthesis of plasmalogens, a special class of membrane phospholipids	Elimination, by the action of catalase, of H_2O_2 generated by the activity of some peroxisomal oxidases
Synthesis of cholesterol and other isoprenoid derivatives, such as dolichol, a complex lipid with an important role in glycoprotein biosynthesis	β-Oxidation of fatty acids, long-chain dicarboxylic acids, the side-chain of cholesterol, and other compounds
Synthesis of bile acids	Oxidation of pipecolic acid, a normally minor intermediate in lysine metabolism
Transamination of glyoxalate to glycine (by the action of alanine:glyoxalate aminotransferase	Spermine and spermidine oxidation

Biochemical studies

The clinical biochemical abnormalities in patients with peroxisomal disorders reflect, to a large extent, the underlying metabolic defects. Defects in peroxisomal biogenesis are, in general, associated with numerous abnormalities, particularly increased levels of very long-chain fatty acids in plasma. Table 9.13 summarizes key laboratory abnormalities in some of the more common peroxisomal disorders.

None of the laboratory investigations shown in Table 9.13 is routine. They are performed primarily in laboratories set up specifically to study peroxisomal disorders.

Plasma very long-chain fatty acids and phytanic acid

The quantitative analysis of very long-chain fatty acids and phytanic acid (a 20-carbon branched-chain fatty acid derived from chlorophyll) requires preliminary extraction and derivatization of complex lipids, followed by preparatory TLC isolation and capillary GC analysis of the fatty acid methyl esters. The analysis is technically challenging, and it is offered by only a small number of specialized laboratories specifically interested in the diagnosis of inborn errors of peroxisomal metabolism.

Table 9.13. *Laboratory abnormalities in some of the peroxisomal disorders.*

Laboratory test	Zellweger syndrome	Ketoacyl-CoA thiolase deficiency	NALD or Infantile Refsum syndrome	XL-ALD	Adult Refsum disease	RCDP
Increased VLCFA	+++	+++	+++	++	–	–
Increased urinary pipecolic acid	+++	+++	++	–	–	–
Decreased red cell plasmalogens	+++	–	++	–	–	+++
Increased plasma phytanic acid	+	–	+ – ++	–	+++	++
Increased plasma bile acid metabolites	+++	+++	+++	–	–	–

Note: NALD, neonatal adrenoleukodystrophy; RCDP, rhizomelic chondrodysplasia punctata; VLCFA, very long-chain fatty acids.

Plasma and urinary pipecolic acid
L-Pipecolic acid is an intermediate in lysine metabolism. Accumulation of the compopund is a characteristic of inherited defects of peroxisome biogenesis. Levels in plasma and urine are normally extremely low. Even in patients with peroxisomal disorders, in whom plasma and urine concentrations may be 100 times normal, the levels are relatively low compared with other diagnostically important biological compounds. After extraction and derivatization, pipecolic acid is usually measured by HPLC, GC, or GC–MS. The sensitivity and accuracy of quantitation is increased by using an isotope-dilution approach to analysis of the compound. Plasma levels may be spuriously elevated in children with hepatocellular disease or by ingestion of vegetables rich in pipecolate.

Red cell plasmalogens
Plasmalogens are major components of the phospholipids of myelin and other membranes, including red cells. Deficiency of plasmalogen biosynthesis in peroxisomal disorders results in decreased concentrations in red cell membranes. Plasmalogens are measured by extraction of membrane lipids and measurement of lipid phosphorus after saponification to remove the phosphoglycerides.

Bibliography
Breningstall, G.N. (1993). Approach to diagnosis of oxidative metabolism disorders. *Pediatric Neurology*, **9**, 81–90.
Chalmers, R. A. & Lawson, A. M. (1982). *Organic Acids in Man.* London: Chapman and Hall Ltd.
Gieselmann, V. (1995). Lysosomal storage diseases. *Biochimica et Biophysica Acta*, **1270**, 103–36.
Hommes, F. A. (Editor), (1991). *Techniques in Diagnostic Human Biochemical Genetics: A Laboratory Manual.* New York: Wiley-Liss, Inc.
Lehotay, D. & Clarke, J. T. R. (1995). Organic acidurias and related abnormalities. *Critical Reviews in Clinical Laboratory Sciences*, **32**, 377–429.
Leroy, J.G., Espeel, M., Gadisseux, J.F., Mandel, H., Martinez, M., Poll-The, B.T., Wanders, R.J.A. & Roels, F. (1995). Diagnostic workup of a peroxisomal patient. In *Diagnosis of Human Peroxisomal Disorders*, ed. F. Roels, S. DeBei, R.B.H. Schutgens & G.T.N. Besley, pp. 214–22. Dordrecht: Kluwer Academic Publishers.
Rustin, P., Chretien, D., Bourgeron, T., Gérard, B., Rötig, A., Saudubray, J.M. & Munnich, A. (1994). Biochemical and molecular investigations in respiratory chain deficiencies. *Clinica Chimica Acta*, **228**, 35–51.
Shoffner, J.M. & Wallace, D.C. (1995). Oxidative phosphorylation diseases. In *The Metabolic and Molecular Bases of Inherited Disease*, 7th edn, ed. C.R. Scriver, A.L. Beaudet, W.S. Sly & D. Valle, pp. 1535–609. New York: McGraw-Hill.
Wallace, D.C. (1992). Diseases of the mitochondrial DNA. *Annual Review of Biochemistry*, **61**, 1175–212.
Wellner, D. & Meister, A. (1981). A survey of inborn errors of amino acid metabolism and transport in man. *Annual Review of Biochemistry*, **50**, 911–68.

10

Treatment

The purpose of this chapter is to present some general principles of the management of inherited metabolic diseases using specific examples to illustrate various points. It is not meant to be a detailed guide to the specific treatment of any particular disease. Instead, it is intended to provide a conceptual scaffold to aid in understanding the strategy behind the management of various inborn errors of metabolism, particularly strategies involving environmental manipulation.

A logical approach to treatment would be to determine how various point defects in metabolism cause disease, and to reverse or neutralize them, either by dietary, pharmacologic, or some other form of metabolic manipulation. However, in many cases, our understanding of how a particular point defect in metabolism produces disease is still incomplete. Often the abnormality is metabolically or physically inaccessible to environmental manipulation. In the discussion to follow, examples are provided of how rational approaches to treatment grew out of an understanding of the primary and secondary consequences of inborn errors of metabolism. The emphasis is on instances in which treatment is at least partially successful.

Control of accumulation of substrate

When disease is caused by accumulation of the substrate of a reaction which is impaired as a result of deficiency of an enzyme of transport protein, a reasonable approach to treatment would be to attempt to control levels of the toxic metabolite either by decreasing its accumulation or accelerating its removal by alternative reactions.

Restricted dietary intake
Phenylketonuria (PKU)
The treatment of PKU by dietary phenylalanine restriction is successful largely because the most obvious clinical abnormalities of the disease are due to

Table 10.1. *Some examples of inborn errors of metabolism treatable by dietary manipulation.*

Disease	Defect	Clinical aspects	Treatment
Disorders of amino acid metabolism			
Phenylketonuria	Phenylalanine hydroxylase	Progressive mental retardation	Phenylalanine restricted diet, possible tyrosine supplementation
Maple syrup urine disease	Branched chain 2-ketoacid decarboxylase	Acute encephalopathy, metabolic acidosis, mental retardation	Diet restricted in leucine, isoleucine, and valine
Homocystinuria	Cystathionine β-synthase	Tall stature, dislocated ocular lens, intravascular thrombosis, mental retardation	Methionine restricted diet, supplemented with vitamin B_6, betaine
Hepatorenal tyrosinemia	Fumarylacetoacetase	Acute liver failure, cirrhosis	Diet restricted in phenylalanine and tyrosine
Lysinuric protein intolerance	Dibasic amino acid transport defect	Acute encephalopathy associated with hyperammonemia	Dietary protein restriction, supplemented with citrulline
Urea cycle enzyme defects	Any of several enzymes involved in urea biosynthesis	Acute encephalopathy associated with hyperammonemia and mental retardation	Dietary protein restriction, supplemented with sodium benzoate, sodium phenylacetate, arginine, citrulline
Disorders of organic acid metabolism			
Methylmalonic acidemia	Methylmalonyl-CoA mutase	Metabolic acidosis, hyperammonemia, and mental retardation	Dietary isoleucine, valine, methionine, and threonine restriction, supplemented with carnitine
Propionic acidemia	Propionyl-CoA carboxylase	Metabolic acidosis, hyperammonemia, and mental retardation	Dietary isoleucine, valine, methionine, and threonine restriction

Isovaleric acidemia	Isovaleryl-CoA dehydrogenase	Metabolic acidosis, hyperammonemia, and mental retardation	Dietary protein restriction, supplemented with carnitine and glycine
Glutaric aciduria, type I	Glutaryl-CoA dehydrogenase	Metabolic acidosis, ataxia	Dietary tryptophan and lysine restriction
Disorders of carbohydrate metabolism			
Galactosemia	Galactose-1-phosphate uridyltransferase	Liver dysfunction, hemolytic anemia, mental retardation	Dietary galactose and lactose restriction
Hereditary fructose intolerance	Fructose-1-phosphate and fructose-6-phosphate aldolase	Hypoglycemia, metabolic acidosis	Dietary fructose and sucrose restriction
Glycogen storage disease, type I	Glucose-6-phosphatase deficiency	Hypoglycemia, lactic acidosis, hyperuricemia	Frequent feeds of glucose or glucose polymer; dietary galactose and fructose restriction
Intestinal disaccharidase deficiencies	Any of several enzymes involved in the digestion of various disaccharides	Chronic diarrhea, failure to thrive	Dietary restriction of disaccharide involved

accumulation of phenylalanine, and ultimately all the phenylalanine in the body is derived from dietary protein. It is not synthesized endogenously. Moreover, it is water soluble, and it equilibrates rapidly among various compartments in the body, including the circulation. In theory, regulation of phenylalanine levels in the body would appear to be relatively easy. However, the practical management of the disease turns out to be somewhat more complicated. Phenylalanine is an essential amino acid. Failure to provide amounts in the diet adequate to support normal protein biosynthesis will result in malnutrition. In some of the original infants with PKU, treated by dietary phenylalanine restriction, this was severe enough to cause their deaths. Most of the phenylalanine in the body by far exists as protein. As such, it is not neurotoxic. However, even subtle shifts in the balance between endogenous protein synthesis and breakdown, such as occur during intercurrent illnesses, can have profound effects on levels of the free amino acid. Marked increases in plasma phenylalanine levels are routinely seen in children with PKU during relatively trivial intercurrent illnesses.

When the conversion of phenylalanine to tyrosine is impaired, as it is in PKU, tyrosine becomes an essential amino acid. PKU diets have generally been considered to contain enough tyrosine to meet the needs for protein, neurotransmitter, and hormone biosynthesis. However, a number of observations on children with PKU suggest that this may not be the case. Some of the suboptimal results of dietary treatment of the disease may be the result of tyrosine deficiency. This is still being examined by many groups of investigators.

In order to avoid inadvertent phenylalanine deficiency, the diets of children with PKU are designed to maintain blood levels of the amino acid two to five times above normal, levels which appear not to be neurotoxic. Although malnutrition and the direct and immediate neurotoxicity of phenylalanine may be avoided in this manner, the increased concentrations of the amino acid interfere with the transport of other amino acids, such as leucine, sharing the same cellular transport systems. The long-term effects of this are unknown.

Despite the theoretical and practical imperfections of the treatment of PKU by dietary phenylalanine restriction, it is the model on which the management of other inborn errors of essential amino acid metabolism is based (Table 10.1).

Galactosemia
Propelled in part by the success experienced with the dietary treatment of PKU, investigators developed a similar strategy for the management of galactosemia. Disease is caused by accumulation of galactose-1-phosphate and, to a lesser extent, galactitol. On the surface, controlling galactose-1-phosphate levels by dietary galactose restriction might appear to be easier than the management of PKU by phenylalanine restriction. It is a significant component of only a limited

number of foods, and it is not essential for adequate nutrition. However, it is synthesized endogenously for use in the synthesis of galactose-containing compounds, such as the myelin lipid, galactocerebroside. The inability to control endogenous biosynthesis limits the extent to which galactose accumulation can be controlled by diet alone. This may be why the outcome of the dietary treatment of the disease is not generally as good as the treatment of PKU.

Many inborn errors of metabolism in which disease is caused by accumulation of a water-soluble metabolite resemble the galactosemia model. In order to be successful, therapeutic strategies must be developed to take into consideration the need to control endogenous production as well as dietary intake of the toxic metabolite. In some cases, this has been achieved by pharmacologic inhibition of endogenous production of the metabolite.

Propionic acidemia

Propionic acidemia, caused by deficiency of propionyl-CoA carboxylase, is characterized by persistent metabolic acidosis as a result of propionic acid accumulation. Treatment is based on controlling propionic acid production by limiting dietary intake of propionic acid precursors: isoleucine, valine, threonine, methionine, thymine, uracil, cholesterol side-chain, and odd-chain fatty acids. The accumulation of the essential amino acids, isoleucine, valine, and threonine, is controllable to some extent by diet. The contribution of dietary and endogenously produced thymine and uracil to propionate accumulation is unknown, but it is probably small. The contribution of the side-chain of cholesterol may be important, and the cholesterol content of therapeutic diets for children with propionic acidemia should be decreased to a minimum.

What sets propionic acidemia and related organic acidopathies (methylmalonic acidemia and isovaleric acidemia) apart from other inborn errors of metabolism is the important contribution of intestinal flora to the accumulation of toxic metabolites. The normal diet contains very small amounts of odd-chain fatty acids, and they are not synthesized endogenously. However, they are produced by intestinal bacteria, which also produce large amounts of propionic acid itself in the gut. These compounds formed in the gut are rapidly absorbed and added to the total body propionic acid pool. Intermittent oral administration of antimicrobials, such as metronidazole, routinely causes a decrease in plasma levels of organic acid.

Control of endogenous production of substrate

Controlling the endogenous production of potentially toxic substrates is a basic aspect of the management of many inherited metabolic diseases. During intercurrent illnesses, patients with amino acidopathies or urea cycle enzyme defects (UCEDs) are routinely treated with high-calorie, nonprotein feeds, taken either orally or intravenously, in an effort to minimize breakdown of body protein. During recovery, amino acids or protein are reintroduced into the diet in a fashion calculated to optimize reparative protein biosynthesis and avoiding starvation-induced catabolism. In the event of acute metabolic decompensation, high-calorie intakes are sometimes combined with infusions of insulin and glucose to further decrease protein breakdown and to promote protein biosynthesis during recovery.

Most of the morbidity associated with inherited fatty acid oxidation defects is preventable by avoiding high fat dietary loads or situations in which the body is required to draw on fat to meet its energy needs. This is achievable by careful adherence to a high-carbohydrate, low-fat diet and sedulous avoidance of fasting. Intervention during intercurrent illnesses should include measures to ensure adequate, uninterrupted delivery of simple carbohydrates, especially glucose, along with fluids and electrolytes. This often requires early consideration of intravenous therapy if the patient is vomiting or otherwise unable to take in adequate amounts of carbohydrate by mouth.

NTBC treatment of hepatorenal tyrosinemia

Disease in hepatorenal tyrosinemia is caused by accumulation of fumarylacetoacetate and maleylacetoacetate, intermediates in the oxidative metabolism of tyrosine. Marked improvement in infants with the disease is often achievable by carefully managed restriction of dietary phenylalanine and tyrosine intakes. However, dietary treatment has generally not arrested some of the more serious complications of the disease, such as recurrent attacks of acute porphyria and the development of cirrhosis and hepatocarcinoma. A major advance in the management of the disease was the introduction of treatment with a drug, 2-(2-nitro-4-trifluoromethylbenzoyl)-1,3-cyclohexanedione (NTBC), which blocks the production of the toxic tyrosine intermediates by inhibiting the enzyme *p*-hydroxyphenylalanine dioxygenase (Figure 10.1).

While it is too early to determine what the overall long-term effects of treatment with NTBC will be, the short-term results have been dramatic in some infants with the disease.

Treatment of X-linked adrenoleukodystrophy with Lorenzo oil

The observation that very long-chain fatty acid (VLCFA) levels are increased in the complex lipids of the brain and many other tissues, including plasma, of patients with X-linked adrenoleukodystrophy (XL–ALD) stimulated efforts to control the disease by dietary restriction of this class of fatty acids, even though

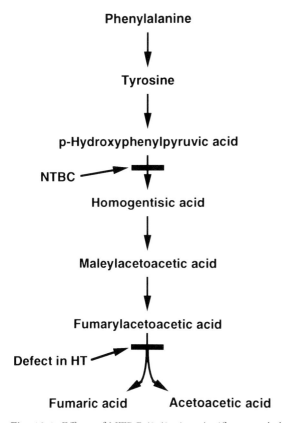

Fig. 10.1. Effects of NTBC (2-(2-nitro-4-trifluoromethylbenzoyl)-1,3-cyclohexane-dione) on tyrosine metabolism.

the relationship between the lipid abnormalities and the development of signs of disease is still not understood. Initial attempts to decrease plasma VLCFA levels by dietary restriction were unsuccessful: endogenous synthesis of the lipids apparently accounted for more than half the VLCFA accumulating in the disease. Subsequent studies on cultured skin fibroblasts showed that endogenous biosynthesis of VLCFA could be inhibited, at least *in vitro*, by treatment with another fatty acid, oleic acid. Studies in patients with XL–ALD showed that supplementation of the low-fat diet with glycerol trioleate (GTO) produces significant improvements in plasma VLCFA levels. However, the effect was incomplete and transient. The addition of erucic acid, another long-chain fatty acid, to the diet resulted in an even greater VLCFA-lowering effect. It is now possible routinely to achieve normal plasma VLCFA levels by treatment of boys with XL–ALD by a low-fat diet supplemented by the mixture of GTO and glycerol trierucate (GTE). The effects of this treatment on disease outcome are still under investigation. The results of preliminary studies suggest that disease onset is delayed significantly in boys in whom treatment is begun pre-symptomatically. Symptomatic boys with the disease and men with ad-renomyeloneuropathy (AMN) do not appear to benefit from the treatment.

Acceleration of removal of substrate
Dialysis (including peritoneal dialysis, hemodialysis, and continuous venous-venous hemofiltration)
One of the most effective methods for the rapid removal of water-soluble toxic substrates is some form of dialysis. Peritoneal dialysis is technically the least demanding. However, it is also the slowest way to remove amino acids, organic acids, or ammonium. Hemodialysis is more rapid, but it is technically very difficult to perform, particularly in neonates, because of the difficulty achieving adequate vascular access. In this respect continuous venous–venous hemofiltra-tion (CVVH) is often preferred because it is generally easier to establish. Exchange transfusion is only effective for short periods of time. As a rule, any patient with an inherited metabolic disease who is considered a candidate for exchange transfusion, as treatment of acute metabolic decompensation, should be dialyzed.

Dialysate volumes and cycling time are probably more important variables in clearing water-soluble metabolites than the pH and composition of the fluid. Nonetheless, an alkaline pH is generally preferred for the optimum clearance of ammonium, and bicarbonate is a better anion than lactate for the treatment of severe metabolic acidosis.

Treatment of UCED with sodium benzoate and sodium phenylacetate
Sodium benzoate is a nontoxic food preservative which is absorbed extremely well from the gut and condenses with glycine to form hippuric acid, which is cleared very efficiently from the circulation by the kidney. Each molecule of hippuric acid formed results in the removal of one atom of waste nitrogen. Sodium phenylacetate is theoretically even more efficient because it condenses rapidly with glutamine to form phenylacetylglutamine, which is excreted taking with it two waste nitrogen atoms per molecule of the drug. Unfortunately, sodium phenylacetate is chemically unstable, and it has a foul odor. Increasingly, it is being replaced by sodium phenylbutyrate, which is more stable, has a less pungent odor, and is converted to phenylacetate in the body. These medications

are particularly useful for the interval control of ammonium levels in patients with UCED, and for the anticipatory management of newborn infants who are at high risk, on the basis of the family history, for having UCED.

Treatment of homocystinuria with betaine

Homocystinuria is an inborn error of the biosynthesis of cystathionine by condensation of the amino acids, homocysteine and serine, a reaction catalyzed by the pyridoxine-requiring enzyme, cystathionine β-synthase (CBS) (see Figure 7.12). Initial efforts to treat the condition focused on measures to decrease the concentration of homocysteine in plasma by limiting endogenous production of the amino acid through dietary methionine restriction. However, the modifications to diet necessary to maintain plasma methionine and homocysteine concentrations at normal levels are difficult and compliance beyond early childhood is generally poor.

In patients who have homocystinuria as a result of CBS deficiency that are not responsive to pharmacologic doses of pyridoxine (discussed later), homocysteine accumulation has been treated by administration of betaine. Betaine promotes methylation of the amino acid to methionine with the production of N,N-dimethylglycine (DMG) in a reaction catalyzed by the enzyme, betaine-homocysteine methyltransferase (Figure 7.12). Treatment causes increased concentrations of methionine, above the already elevated levels occurring in untreated patients with homocystinuria. This has been a matter of some concern because methionine is toxic to the liver, at least in experimental animals. Nevertheless, betaine treatment is widely used in an effort to control the complications of homocysteine accumulation in patients with CBS deficiency that is not responsive to pyridoxine therapy.

Treatment of organic acidopathies with carnitine or glycine

In many of the inborn errors of metabolism, the substrate of the reaction affected is the coenzyme A ester of one or more low molecular weight organic acids, such as propionic acid or methylmalonic acid. Accumulation of the compounds sequesters coenzyme A making it unavailable for other important processes and reactions in which it plays a central role. These include a critical role in fatty acid oxidation (see Chapter 5), fatty acid biosynthesis, pyruvate oxidation (see Chapter 4), and a vast assortment of biological acetylations. One of the latter is acetylation of glutamate, a reaction catalyzed by N-acetylglutamate synthetase, which is required for the activation of carbamylphosphate synthase I, the first reaction in urea biosynthesis. One of the important secondary metabolic consequences of organic acid accumulation is hyperammonemia, which appears to be caused by impaired ureagenesis resulting from insufficiency of *N*-acetylglutamate.

Transesterification of organic acyl-CoA esters, with the release of free coenzyme A, appears to be one of the important roles of carnitine. The formation of organic acylcarnitines not only restores free coenzyme A levels, it facilitates excretion of the organic acids because the renal clearance of acylcarnitines is greater than that of the free acids. This is the reason why accumulation of organic acids, including many drugs, ultimately causes carnitine depletion. It is also why analysis of urinary or plasma acylcarnitines by gas chromatography–mass spectrometry (see Chapter 9) is helpful in the diagnosis of inborn errors of organic acid metabolism. Treatment of organic acidopathies with carnitine is an important adjunct to the dietary management of the diseases. It restores tissue carnitine concentrations for use in processes like the transport of fatty acids into mitochondria (see Chapter 5). Carnitine treatment also contributes to ensuring adequate supplies of free coenzyme A, and it facilitates removal of toxic organic acid metabolites.

Some organic acids condense readily with glycine to form acylglycine esters. In the case of isovaleric acidemia, most of the isovaleric acid recovered in urine occurs as isovalerylglycine. The alacrity with which this occurs is exploited to enhance excretion of accumulated organic acid in the urine by treating affected patients with large oral doses of glycine.

Replacement of product

Replacement of the reaction product is the most logical approach to the management of inherited metabolic diseases in which the symptoms of disease are due to deficiency of the product. For example, this would apply to all the disorders of hormone biosynthesis. However, it also applies to metabolic situations in which intermediary metabolites become sequestrated as a result of defects in membrane transport.

Reaction product replacement
Thyroid treatment of congenital goitrous hypothyroidism
The treatment of inborn errors of thyroid hormone biosynthesis is not fundamentally different from the treatment of athyrotic hypothyroidism. Administration of thyroid hormone is all that is needed to control symptoms arising as a result of thyroid hormone deficiency.

Treatment of hyperammonemia-hyperornithinemia-homocitrullinemia (HHH)
syndrome with ornithine

Most of the symptoms and disability associated with HHH syndrome are the result of chronic and acute-on-chronic hyperammonemia due to intramitochondrial ornithine deficiency caused by an inborn error of mitochondrial ornithine transport. Plasma ornithine concentrations in affected patients are elevated. However, a low-protein diet supplemented with pharmacologic amounts of L-ornithine greatly enhances urea biosynthesis by forcing ornithine into mitochondria where it is needed to condense with carbamylphosphate to form citrulline (see Figure 2.5). This approach to management of the disease is not without some risk: excess intramitochondrial ornithine is probably what causes the ocular problems in patients with gyrate atrophy caused by intramitochondrial ornithine transaminase deficiency.

Treatment of argininosuccinic aciduria (ASAuria) with arginine

The hyperammonemia in patients with ASAuria is due to intramitochondrial ornithine deficiency, which is, in turn, due to deficiency of arginine from which ornithine is formed by enzymic elimination of urea. Argininosuccinate lyase (AL) deficiency blocks the formation of arginine by AL-catalyzed elimination of fumaric acid (see Figure 2.5). Treatment of the acute hyperammonemia in patients with ASAuria by administration of arginine, either as the hydrochloride or the free base, results in dramatic resolution of the hyperammonemia. It is because the response to treatment of this disease by administration of arginine is so dramatic that patients with newly recognized, symptomatic hyperammonemia should be treated with intravenous arginine hydrochloride immediately the possibility of a UCED is considered. It may be live-saving.

Gene product replacement

In many inherited metabolic diseases, disease-producing accumulation of substrate is not affected by dietary manipulation or conventional pharmacologic interventions. This is the case, for example, with all the lysosomal storage disorders. The lysosomal breakdown of complex carbohydrates and lipids is a constitutive degradative process which is not significantly influenced by practical environmental manipulations. However, the relatively indiscriminant uptake of 'foreign' proteins into secondary lysosomes by the process of endocytosis has been exploited in the development of enzyme replacement strategies for the management of at some of these diseases.

Lysosomal enzymes are synthesized in the rough endoplasmic reticulum like other proteins. In the course biosynthesis, they are glycosylated by a complex co-translational process, followed by specific modifications of the oligosaccharide in the Golgi apparatus which produce a recognition signal for targeting the nascent enzyme glycoprotein to primary lysosomes. This involves the production of mannose-6-phosphate residues which bind specific receptors in lysosomal membranes. Inside primary lysosomes, further proteolytic modification of the pro-enzyme polypeptide occurs, and the mannose phosphate residues are removed. Similar systems of receptor-mediated binding and uptake of lysosomal enzymes exist at the cell surface. As a result, lysosomal enzymes infused into the circulation tend to be taken up by cells of various types and to become localized in lysosomes, precisely where they would normally become localized for the metabolism of complex, water-insoluble compounds, such as glycosphingolipids.

Although numerous attempts have been made to treat various lysosomal storage diseases by enzyme replacement, success has been limited by shortages of suitably purified enzymes, adverse allergic reactions, and the inaccessibility of the target tissue, particularly brain, to infused enzyme. Nevertheless, this remains one of the most promising areas of research into treatment on lysosomal storage diseases in which the brain is not involved.

Alglucerase treatment of Gaucher disease

The successful treatment of Gaucher disease by infusions of 'engineered' human glucocerebrosidase represents a major milestone in the management of inherited metabolic diseases. Glucocerebroside extracted and purified from pooled human placenta, or produced now by recombinant DNA technology, is enzymically modified to remove the terminal sialic acid, galactose, and N-acetylglucosamine residues from the glycoprotein oligosaccharide, a process which was shown to greatly enhance uptake by tissue macrophages by exposing mannose residues involved in receptor-mediated uptake of the enzyme. Intravenous infusion of adequate doses of suitably modified enzyme, called alglucerase, as infrequently as every two to four weeks produces a dramatic decrease in spleen size and improvements of hemoglobin and platelet counts in patients with Gaucher disease within a few months. The bone lesions are slower to respond to enzyme replacement treatment. Enzyme replacement may delay, but does not prevent, the onset of neurologic symptoms in patients with acute neuronopathic Gaucher disease (type II); the effect on neurologic symptoms in patients with subacute disease, called type III, has not yet been determined.

Adverse reactions to alglucerase treatment are rare and almost always mild. Unfortunately, expansion of the use of enzyme replacement therapy for severe non-neuronopathic Gaucher disease has been limited, not by concerns about its efficacy or safety, but by its enormous cost. The cost of the first year of treatment of an average adult with the disease could easily exceed $250,000 US.

Cofactor replacement therapy

The catalytic properties of many enzymes depend on the participation of non-protein prosthetic groups, such as vitamins or minerals, as obligatory cofactors. In fact, the nutritional value of vitamins stems largely from their role as catalytically important prosthetic groups of specific enzymes (Table 10.2).

Nutritional vitamin deficiency affects most or all enzymatic reactions in which the particular vitamin plays a role as a prosthetic group. The clinical effects of nutritional vitamin deficiency cannot always be traced to the effect of the deficiency one specific enzyme. Treatment of diseases caused by nutritional vitamin deficiencies by administration of amounts of the relevant vitamin only five to ten times higher than the amounts present in a normal diet generally results in rapid resolution of the symptoms of deficiency, though the effects of secondary tissue damage may persist.

Defects in the absorption of specific vitamins or mineral cofactors may have widespread metabolic effects similar to those produced by dietary cofactor deficiency. In some cases, the cause of the malabsorption can be traced to a genetic defect in intestinal or renal uptake due to mutations affecting a specific receptor required for transport of the cofactor across the intestinal or renal epithelium. Whether the vitamin or cofactor deficiency is due to malabsorption resulting from acquired disease or to a mutation affecting receptor function, the effect and the response to therapy is the same. The symptoms of deficiency are generally indistinguishable from those caused by dietary deficiency of the specific vitamin. Moreover, treatment with relatively small amounts of the vitamin, administered by injection, to circumvent the barrier of the intestinal mucosa, generally results in rapid resolution of the symptoms of deficiency. An example of this type of problem is anemia due to defects in the intestinal absorption of vitamin B_{12}. Treatment with injections of as little as 1 mg of vitamin B_{12} per month is generally sufficient to prevent the development of symptoms of deficiency.

Disease may also arise as a result of mutations affecting the normal metabolic processing of a vitamin or cofactor. For example, one form of vitamin D-dependent rickets is caused by deficiency of the enzyme which converts the relatively inactive vitamin precursor, 25-hydroxycholecalciferol, to fully active 1α,25-dihydroxycholecalciferol. The clinical effects are indistinguishable from severe nutritional vitamin D deficiency. Treatment with very large doses of

Table 10.2. *Various cofactors involved in intermediary metabolism and implicated in some cofactor-responsive inborn errors of metabolism.*

Cofactor	Function	Cofactor responsive disorders
Thiamine (Vitamin B$_1$)	Reactions involving transfers of acetate groups (e.g. transaldolase, transketolase)	Some cases of lactic acidosis due to pyruvate dehydrogenase deficiency Thiamine-responsive megaloblastic anemia-diabetes-deafness Rare cases of maple syrup urine disease
Riboflavin (Vitamin B$_2$)	Oxidation and reduction reactions	Some cases of multiple acyl-CoA dehydrogenase deficiency (glutaric aciduria, type II)
Pyridoxine (Vitamin B$_6$)	Transaminations, decarboxylations, rearrangements of many amino acids	About 50% of cases of homocystinuria due to cystathionine β-synthase deficiency Pyridoxine-responsive seizures of infancy Cystathioninuria Xanthurenic aciduria Hyperornithinemia with gyrate atrophy
Cobalamin (Vitamin B$_{12}$)	Methyl group (–CH$_3$) transfer reactions	Methylmalonic acidemia (*cblA*, *cblB*) Homocystinuria and methylmalonic aciduria (*cblC*, *cblD*, *cblF*) Some cases of homocystinuria (*cblE*, *cblG*)
Folic acid	One-carbon metabolism, particularly in nucleic acid synthesis	Some cases of homocystinuria
Ascorbic acid (Vitamin C)	Hydroxylation of proline and lysine in collagen synthesis; enzymic conversion of *p*-hydroxyphenylpyruvic acid to homogentisic acid	Some disorders of mitochondrial electron transport (unproven)

Biotin	Reactions involving chemical transfers of CO_2 (e.g. pyruvate carboxylase, acetyl-CoA carboxylase)	Biotinidase deficiency
Vitamin K	Carboxylation of glutamate residues of proteins of the blood clotting system	Some disorders of mitochondrial electron transport (unproven)
Cholecalciferol (Vitamin D)	Calcium absorption and mineralization of bone	Vitamin D-dependent rickets
Pantothenic acid	Functions as acyl group carrier in fatty acid metabolism (as part of Coenzyme A)	
Nicotinamide	Oxidation and reduction reactions throughout metabolism	Hartnup disease
Coenzyme Q_{10}	Mitochondrial electron transport	Some disorders of mitochondrial electron transport (unproven)
Lipoic acid	Oxidation, reduction and acyl transfer reactions (e.g. pyruvate dehydrogenase)	Some cases of pyruvate dehydrogenase deficiency

vitamin precursor or physiologic doses of the active vitamin produces rapid resolution of the symptoms of disease.

Disease may also occur as a result of mutations in the enzyme protein affecting the utilization or binding of the vitamin or mineral cofactor. In these cases, the effect of the defect is specific and limited to the reaction catalyzed by the mutant enzyme protein. In cases like this, the outcome is often clinically indistinguishable from the effects of mutations involving any other site in the enzyme protein affecting its catalytic properties. Treatment of disease caused by mutations affecting vitamin or cofactor utilization with amounts of the cofactor several hundred times the dosages generally required to prevent the development of symptoms of nutritional deficiency often results in correction of the metabolic defect and reversal of the signs of disease. Because the metabolic abnormality is confined to a single reaction, among the many in which the cofactor may be involved, and reversal of symptoms requires very large doses of cofactor, these conditions have been called vitamin or cofactor dependencies to distinguish them from the more generalized metabolic effects of nutritional deficiencies which are, moreover, correctable by low doses of the relevant vitamin or cofactor. Table 10.2 shows several examples of vitamin responsive inborn errors of metabolism.

Pyridoxine-responsive homocystinuria

CBS requires pyridoxine as a prosthetic group for catalytic activity. In about half the patients with CBS-deficiency homocystinuria, methionine and homocystine levels in plasma are decreased to normal, and thromboembolic complications of the disease are prevented, by administration of vitamin B_6 (pyridoxine), in dosages (250 to 500 mg per day) far in excess of those necessary to prevent clinical pyridoxine deficiency in otherwise healthy humans. The catalytically active form of vitamin B_6 is pyridoxal phosphate, derived from the metabolism of dietary pyridoxal, pyridoxine, and pyridoxamine. In the course of the CBS-catalyzed reaction of serine with homocysteine, a covalently bound pyridoxal-homocysteine intermediate is formed followed by rapid condensation with serine and release of the pyridoxal aldehyde group. Pyridoxal phosphate is tightly bound by noncovalent interactions with amino acids at the active site of the apoenzyme protein. The specificity and affinity of binding are determined by the amino acid sequence of the active site which is determined by the nucleotide sequence of the CBS gene. Pyridoxine responsiveness in some patients with homocystinuria has been shown to be caused by a decrease in the affinity of pyridoxal phosphate binding by the mutant apoenzyme with the result that the production of active holoenzyme is insufficient to control accumulation of the amino acid.

Vitamin B₁₂-responsive methylmalonic acidemia

Vitamin B$_{12}$-responsive methylmalonic acidemia

Methylmalonic acidemia is caused by deficiency of the mitochondrial cobala-min-dependent enzyme, methylmalonyl-CoA mutase (mut). The resulting accumulation of methylmalonyl-CoA in tissues often causes severe metabolic acidosis due to accumulation of methylmalonic acid (see Chapter 4).

Several genetically distinct forms of mut deficiency have been described. Mutations of the apoenzyme resulting in total deficiency of enzyme activity, designated *mut⁰*, are associated with clinically severe disease. Other mut mutations are characterized by impaired holoenzyme biosynthesis owing to decreased affinity of the apoenzyme for the obligatory cofactor, adenosyl-cobalamin. Disease caused by this type of mutation, designated *mut⁻*, is generally clinically milder and often responds metabolically and clinically to treatment with very large doses of vitamin B$_{12}$ (e.g. 1 mg per day by injection).

By the application of genetic complementation analyses using cultured skin fibroblasts, a number of genetically distinct defects in cobalamin metabolism have been identified in patients with methylmalonic acidemia (see Figure 4.6). *CblA* and *cblB* mutations are both characterized by defects in adenosylcobalamin biosynthesis, and the resulting diseases are clinically indistinguishable at presentation. However, patients with *cblA* defects respond, at least initially, to treatment with large doses of vitamin B$_{12}$; the response of patients with *cblB* disease to vitamin therapy is poor.

Biotin-responsive multiple carboxylase deficiency

Biotin participates as an obligatory cofactor in four carboxylase-catalyzed reactions: acetyl-CoA carboxylase, propionyl-CoA carboxylase, pyruvate car-boxylase, and 3-methylcrotonyl-CoA carboxylase. In each case, the cofactor is bound covalently to the apoenzyme in a reaction catalyzed by the enzyme, holocarboxylase synthetase. Biotin is salvaged during the course of normal enzyme protein degradation by a reaction catalyzed by another enzyme, biotinidase. Deficiency of either holocarboxylase synthetase or biotinidase causes combined deficiency of all four carboxylases. In the first case, deficiency of holocarboxylase synthetase results in failure to form the required active holoenzymes. In the second, failure to hydrolyze the biotin from the degraded enzyme proteins ultimately results in loss of the cofactor by excretion as a protein breakdown product, producing systemic biotin deficiency. In both conditions, the response to treatment with relatively low doses (10–20 mg per day) of oral biotin is often dramatic.

Mitochondrial electron transport defects

Mitochondrial electron transport involves the participation of a number of low molecular weight, nonprotein cofactors, such as flavins, nicotinamide, ubiquinone, iron-sulfur clusters, and heme. Moreover, many compounds not normally involved in mitochondrial electron transport may function as electron transporters under special circumstances. Experience with other systems in which nonprotein cofactors are involved has stimulated attempts to treat mitochondrial electron transport defects with pharmacological dosages of the various prosthetic groups normally implicated in the transport process, or by administration of other electron acceptors, such as ascorbate or various vitamin K derivatives (e.g., menadione, phylloquinone).

Another approach currently being explored by various investigators is to decrease reliance on electron transport via Complex I by enhancing Complex II activity. This is done by treating the patient with large doses of succinate. The rationale might be better understood by reference to Figure 4.3.

Dichloroacetate has been used with some success to treat lactic acidosis of various sorts, including that associated with some inherited metabolic diseases. It acts by inhibiting pyruvate dehydrogenase (PDH) kinase and thereby preventing phosphorylation-mediated inactivation of PDH. What place it has in the treatment of mitochondrial electron transport chain (ETC) defects has yet to be determined.

In spite of scattered reports of beneficial results with these and other approaches to the treatment of mitochondrial ETC defects, none appears to work consistently or well in any predictable way. This is an area of metabolism that clearly requires careful clinical investigation involving collaboration among many centers to accumulate sufficient numbers of patients to evaluate confidently the results of therapy.

Gene transfer therapy

The ultimate treatment of single gene disorders would be to replace the disease-producing mutant gene with a normal gene in a fashion that would ensure long-term, normally regulated expression in the tissues and organs affected by the disease. Although this might be theoretically possible by germ cell gene transfer, the risks associated with this form of treatment are generally considered to be unacceptable. Most attention on gene transfer therapies in humans has focused on treatment of somatic cells. The goal of therapy is to achieve the incorporation and expression of sufficient amounts of normal genetic material in appropriate tissues to achieve long-term correction of the genetic defect. This has been approached in two quite different ways.

Organ transplantation

Many primary genetic diseases have been 'cured' by replacement of the entire organ in which expression of the mutant gene causes disease. This is a rather indiscriminant form of gene transfer therapy, for not only is the disease-producing mutant gene replaced, but every other gene in the tissue is replaced as well. One condition in which this has been successful is hepatorenal tyrosinemia. With the possible exception of the renal tubular dysfunction, the clinical manifestations of the disease are attributable almost entirely to the effect the mutation has on the liver. Liver transplantation is virtually curative.

Bone marrow transplantation (BMT) is another form of gene transfer therapy achieved by organ transplantation. This approach to gene transfer therapy has been used with success in the management of inherited metabolic disorders of hematopoietic tissues, such as severe combined immunodeficiency (SCID) caused by adenosine deaminase (ADA) deficiency. The principle is the same as that applying in the treatment of hepatorenal tyrosinemia by liver transplantation. However, in another group of diseases which do not significantly affect hematopoietic tissues, BMT is being employed as a vehicle for delivering gene product to other tissues in the body. This approach is being aggressively evaluated for the treatment of various lysosomal storage diseases, such as the mucopolysaccharidoses. BMT in most of these disorders is regarded primarily as an enzyme factory. Donor enzyme may work only locally to catalyze the metabolism of substrate brought to it, or it may be secreted into the circulation and taken up by host tissues throughout the body. More experience is required with this approach to treatment to determine its place in the long-term management of inherited metabolic diseases.

Single gene transfer therapy

All single gene transfer therapy of inherited metabolic diseases is still regarded as experimental. The approach that seems to offer the most promise at present is *ex vivo*, retrovirus-mediated gene transfer into hematopoietic stem cells for the management of diseases primarily affecting blood cells or blood cell derivatives. Clinical protocols have been approved for the evaluation of this approach to the treatment of ADA deficiency and of Gaucher disease. Protocols have also been approved for the evaluation of a similar *ex vivo* retrovirus-mediated gene transfer approach to the treatment of homozygous familial hypercholesterolemia. In this condition, liver is obtained from the patient by open biopsy, and cultured hepatocytes are transduced *ex vivo* with normal LDL receptor cDNA and infused back into the portal vein anticipating they will become engrafted and the transgene expressed in the host liver.

Bibliography

Barton, N.W., Brady, R.O., Dambrosia, J.M., Di Bisceglie, A.M., Doppelt, S.H., Hill, S.C., Makin, H.J., Murray, G.J., Parker, R.I., Argoff, C.E., Grewal, R.P. & Yu, K.-T. (1991). Replacement therapy for inherited enzyme deficiency – macrophage-targeted glucocerebrosidase for Gaucher's disease. *New England Journal of Medicine*, 324, 1464–70.

Brusilow, S.W. (1991). Treatment of urea cycle disorders. In *Treatment of Genetic Diseases*, ed. R.J. Desnick, pp. 79–94. New York: Churchill-Livingstone.

Krivit, W. & Shapiro, E.G. (1991). Bone marrow transplantation for storage diseases. In *Treatment of Genetic Diseases*, ed. R.J. Desnick, pp. 203–22. New York: Churchill-Livingstone.

Levy, H.L. (1991). Nutritional therapy in inborn errors of metabolism. In *Treatment of Genetic Diseases*, ed. R.J. Desnick, pp. 1–22. New York: Churchill-Livingstone.

Moser, H.W. & Borel, J. (1995). Dietary management of X-linked adrenoleukodystrophy. *Annual Review of Nutrition*, 15, 379–97.

Parker, P.H., Ballen, M. & Greene, H.L. (1993). Nutritional management of glycogen storage disease. *Annual Review of Nutrition*, 13, 83–109.

Przyrembel, H. (1987). Therapy of mitochondrial disorders. *Journal of Inherited Metabolic Disease*, 10, 129–46.

Thompson, G.N., Butt, W.W., Shann, F.A., Kirby, D.M., Henning, R.D., Howells, D.W. & Osborne, A. (1991). Continuous venovenous hemofiltration in the management of acute decompensation in inborn errors of metabolism. *Journal of Pediatrics*, 118, 879–84.

Index